Prescription for the People

A volume in the series
THE CULTURE AND POLITICS OF HEALTH CARE WORK

Edited by Suzanne Gordon and Sioban Nelson

For a list of titles in the series, visit our website at cornellpress.cornell.edu.

PRESCRIPTION FOR THE PEOPLE

An Activist's Guide to Making Medicine Affordable for All

FRAN QUIGLEY

ILR PRESS
AN IMPRINT OF
CORNELL UNIVERSITY PRESS
ITHACA AND LONDON

First published 2017 by Cornell University Press

Printed in the United States of America

Library of Congress Cataloging-in-Publication Data

Names: Quigley, Fran, 1962– author.
Title: Prescription for the people : an activist's guide to making medicine
    affordable for all / Fran Quigley.
Description: Ithaca : ILR Press, an imprint of Cornell University Press,
    2017. | Series: The culture and politics of health care work | Includes
    bibliographical references and index.
Identifiers: LCCN 2017020499 (print) | LCCN 2017022718 (ebook) |
    ISBN 9781501713927 (epub/mobi) | ISBN 9781501713910 (pdf) |
    ISBN 9781501713750 (pbk. : alk. paper)
Subjects: LCSH: Drugs—Prices—United States. | Prescription pricing—
    United States. | Drug accessibility—United States. | Pharmaceutical
    policy—United States. | Pharmaceutical industry—United States. |
    Health care reform—United States.
Classification: LCC HD9666.4 (ebook) | LCC HD9666.4 .Q54 2017
    (print) | DDC 338.4/36150973—dc23
LC record available at https://lccn.loc.gov/2017020499

Cornell University Press strives to use environmentally responsible
suppliers and materials to the fullest extent possible in the publishing
of its books. Such materials include vegetable-based, low-VOC inks
and acid-free papers that are recycled, totally chlorine-free, or partly
composed of nonwood fibers. For further information, visit our website
at cornellpress.cornell.edu.

To Ellen

CONTENTS

Acknowledgments

Over the years, I have had many opportunities to be an advocate, writer, and teacher connected to important human rights efforts. But I am fairly new to the struggle for access to medicines. My ignorance has one advantage: I have been able to see the campaign for medicine access through an outsider's eyes. Often, those eyes have stared in bewilderment at the thick layers of complexity and technical language that obscure the core claim of the campaign: access to medicines is a moral imperative and a human right.

Those layers of complexity are applied by defenders of the status quo, who are happy to intimidate the rest of us into throwing up our hands in frustration. But more seasoned advocates confess that they too can lapse into relying on technical vocabulary and little-known references. My hope is that this book serves to dismantle much of that intimidating barrier.

As you may imagine, my ignorance also brought significant disadvantages to this project. I have had a lot to learn. The extent to which I have been able to overcome those disadvantages is to the credit of five groups of people.

The first group is represented in the extensive endnotes. This brief, straightforward book is built on hundreds of references to more in-depth work by others. Those scholars, activists and patients were my teachers in a self-study access-to-medicines master class. They are all deserving of my thanks and of the thanks of all of us who care about increasing access to essential medicines. Some of the most prolific and incisive writers on this topic deserve special recognition, especially Ellen t'Hoen, James Love, and Brook Baker.

The second group consists of the dozens of access-to-medicines experts who carved precious time out of their hectic schedules for conversations or interviews with me. Some of the interviews led directly to parts of this book, and all helped provide the background for its content. So, my heart-felt thanks goes to, in alphabetical order, Malini Aisola, Alejandra Alayza, Keaton Andreas, Brook Baker, Stephanie Burgos, Krista Cox, the late Tobeka Daki, Sophie Delaunay, Al Engelberg, Andrew Goldman, Linda Greef, Ethan Guillen, Zahara Heckscher, Julia Hill, Jordan Jarvis, Joanna Keenan, Rachel Kiddell-Monroe, Sandeep Kishore, Stephen Lewis, Javier Llamoza, James Love, Marcus Low, Hannah Lyon, Luz Marina Umbasia, Manuel Martin, Mary-Jane Matsolo, Peter Maybarduk, Fifa Rahman, Manon Ress, Judit Rius Sanjuan, Claudio Ruiz, Zack Struver, Catherine Tomlinson, Els Torreele, and Heba Wanis.

The third group are the Indiana University McKinney School of Law students who contributed their talents in researching, checking sources, and offering feedback on various portions of the book. Sarah Asrar conducted interviews with medicine activists in India and helped write an article based on that experience. Darwinson Valdez interpreted for several interviews. Jessie Howenstine deserves particular thanks because she spent many hours cleaning up the endnote references and offered insightful and very helpful comments on various drafts of this book. Jessie, Chris Stack, M.D., and my sister, Katy Quigley, were inspiring sources of much-appreciated enthusiasm for this book and the cause it promotes.

The fourth group includes Jessie and others who gave their time to read all or parts of this book in draft form and then offered suggestions that significantly improved what you are reading now. Those readers include Katy Quigley, Peter Maybarduk, and Bob Healey. I am very grateful to both for the hours spent reading and providing honest and supportive feedback. Carmel Williams, executive editor of the *Health and Human Rights*

Journal, published my first-ever in-depth piece on access to medicines and subsequent articles, and she both provided encouragement and suggested paths to better writing on this topic. Suzanne Gordon enthusiastically supported this book and called on her extensive experience in health advocacy, health care, and journalism to consistently provide guidance that made each draft better than the last. As always, Ellen White Quigley was my first and most trusted reader and editor.

The final group deserving of acknowledgement here has formed the core of this and every other project I ever have or will undertake. With Sam, Katie, and Jack, I have been enormously blessed with children who are kind, super-smart, and funny. That means they take after their mother, of course. This book is dedicated to her. Ellen provides a bottomless spring of love, patience, wisdom, and support far beyond anything I could ever deserve.

PRESCRIPTION FOR THE PEOPLE

INTRODUCTION

The high cost of essential medicines is a big problem. Recently, here in the United States where I live, social media and even lawmakers exploded in anger over a 400 percent-plus increase in the lifesaving allergy medicine EpiPen. Similar outrage occurred when a young pharmaceutical corporation chief executive officer (CEO) increased the price of a critical toxoplasmosis drug by more than 5,000 percent overnight—just because he could. A hundred-plus cancer physicians took to the pages of the prestigious journal *Mayo Clinic Proceedings* to write an impassioned article decrying the greed of the pharmaceutical industry. These physicians complained that drug companies were setting medicine prices so high that one out of every five of their patients was unable to fill his or her prescriptions. In response to all these incidents and the popular outrage they have inspired, patients, caregivers, and politicians from both major political parties have leveled charges of medicine price gouging against the pharmaceutical companies.

Even for those of us who are fortunate enough to not be poor and to have health insurance, the cost of medicines has a big impact. The cost of medicines drains the budgets of our governments, and barriers to accessing medicines lead to more expensive health care treatments and illnesses that drag down our economy. Polls show that three-quarters of Americans believe that drug costs are unreasonable and that those prices reflect the greed of drug companies.[1]

For the poor and the uninsured, access to medicines is a matter of life and death. Millions of people need medicines that are priced at levels they simply cannot afford. These suffering patients face a real problem: their desperate need for affordable drugs clashes with the core business model of a powerful industry.

On one side of that clash are multinational pharmaceutical corporations, which make up one of the most profitable and politically influential industries in history. That industry is determined to protect monopoly prices on patented medicines. On the other side of the clash are the sick and the poor, joined by advocates scattered across the globe in small, usually underfunded organizations. At first glance, it doesn't seem like a fair fight. But patients and medicine activists have won before.

In the midst of the HIV/AIDS crisis of the late 1990s and early 2000s, millions of people were dying because they could not afford lifesaving drugs. Patients and activists who wanted to change this tragic reality faced fierce resistance from a formidable collaboration between Big Pharma and the U.S. government. The multinational corporations and the world's economic superpower were intent on preserving the high monopoly price tags on patented AIDS drugs and to block affordable generic alternatives. But the activists working in the United States, sub-Saharan Africa, South America, and Asia pushed back hard. They flooded the streets with protests, filed lawsuits, and mercilessly heckled the drug companies and politicians. They made a moral claim that medicine should be for people, not profits, and that there is a fundamental human right to essential medicines. That message resonated across the world, and these activists eventually triumphed, reducing the costs of the medicines by as much as 99 percent; setting the stage for a massive global distribution of the drugs. Millions of lives were saved.

But the fruits of that victory, the widespread availability of cheap HIV/AIDS medicines, is an exception to the rule. Whereas millions once died of untreated HIV/AIDS, now millions die from untreated cancer. Children die because their families cannot afford vaccinations. The episodic drug pricing outrages, such as the reaction to the EpiPen price hike or the overreach of the "Pharma Bro" Martin Shkreli, have not led to systemic change.

So the same activists who pushed for HIV/AIDS treatment, accompanied by a new generation of advocates, are trying to produce a sequel with an even more ambitious script than they followed at the turn of the century. Their aim is to make all essential drugs accessible by reclaiming medicines as a public good instead of a profit-making commodity.

One of these activists' biggest challenges is that the terms of their fight can seem complex and confusing. Too often, calls for reform get bogged down in technical intellectual property terms—*compulsory licensing, data exclusivity,* and *patent linkage*—and confusing acronyms for international trade agreements—TRIPS (Trade-Related Aspects of Intellectual Property Rights Agreement), TRIPS-Plus, and TPP (Trans-Pacific Partnership Agreement). This thicket of complexity provides cover for corporations that rely on the for-profit medicine model and are determined to protect the status quo. As one leading medicine activist admitted to me, "The problem we have is that there are only a handful of people in the world who know what we are taking about."[2]

It does not have to be this way. My aim in this book is to help clear away for you the thicket of jargon that surrounds this crisis so that you can effectively argue for a complete shift in the global approach to developing and providing essential medicines. This shift would restore the longtime historical recognition that medicines are a public good, reflecting the global consensus that access to essential medicines is a human right.

Because every cure starts with an accurate diagnosis, in this book I explain how and why the current medicines system is dysfunctional and corrupt. We all want both affordable medicines and innovation in research and development, so I explain the proven approaches to accomplishing that balance. Most of us reject the status quo of corporations making record-breaking profits on medicines that are priced out of the range of the sick and the dying, so I set out the moral and rights-based foundation of the case for universal access to medicines. Finally, if you want to take action and speak out for access to medicines—and I sincerely hope you do—the conclusion to this book is devoted to helping you get started.

I chose to structure the book around twenty-two arguments for why we must reform our medicines system and how to do so. Each chapter contains a single argument. I encourage you to skim the table of contents both before you read the book and afterward. When you need to refer to a particular issue connected with access to medicines—such as the fruits of government-funded medicines research being handed over to corporations for profit-making (chapters 14 and 15)—the table of contents will guide you.

This book is a short one. At the same time, all the points I make here are thoroughly sourced. Many, many researchers and activists have written important detailed analyses of these issues; so you will see hundreds of notes to prior work that backs up the arguments I make here. I have placed those sources in endnotes at the end of the book so you can read the main text without interruption, if you wish.

My hope is that this book will serve as a primer for all who are concerned about access to medicines. My hope is also that this book will buttress the analyses of researchers and the arguments of activists. Most important, my hope is that this book will help you become informed and prepared to play your role in the life and death struggle for access to medicines.

Part I

TOXIC IMPACTS

1

PEOPLE EVERYWHERE ARE STRUGGLING TO GET THE MEDICINES THEY NEED

Hannah Lyon was just twenty-six years old when she was diagnosed with advanced cervical cancer.[1] To her first set of doctors, Lyon's best-case scenario was chemotherapy and radiation that would extend her life for only a few years. Desperate for a more promising approach, Lyon found a clinical trial at the National Institutes of Health (NIH). There she received cutting-edge immunotherapy, in which her immune cells were removed, genetically modified, and reinserted into her bloodstream. Since the treatment, Lyon's tumors have shrunk more than 80 percent.

But Lyon soon realized that most cancer patients are not so fortunate. She saw fellow patients struggling to pay for the medicines that were their only hope for survival. Lyon learned that others had simply been unable to pay and therefore had died from highly treatable cancers.

Lyon had heard the pharmaceutical industry argument that the high medicine prices are necessary to fund drug research. But, then, during her own treatment at the government-funded NIH, Lyon noticed something. "When I had my cell infusion, there were pharmaceutical reps in the room, because they want to take that treatment and offer it commercially. So this whole argument that pharma corporations need long monopoly periods to pay for the research . . . well, they are not even the ones *doing* the research! They did not develop that drug. They are just going to take that drug and charge people tons of money."

Lyon began reading about medicine patents and the international trade agreements that protect them. She learned how government-funded research, not corporate investment, is the most important driver in creating new medicines. She discovered that our profit-driven medicines system is neglecting development of lifesaving medicines in favor of lucrative drugs to address hair loss or sexual performance.

Then Lyon happened to see a television interview with Zahara Heckscher, a breast cancer patient who had been arrested while protesting at the Trans-Pacific Partnership Agreement (TPP) negotiations in Atlanta in October 2015. The TPP was the latest in a series of trade deals that proposed to lock in corporate medicine monopolies and lock out suffering patients from the treatment they need. As we learn in chapter 18, the TPP promised to be particularly damaging to patients who need the kind of cutting-edge treatment that both Hannah Lyon and Zahara Heckscher received. So Heckscher had decided to use her status as a cancer patient to raise awareness of the dysfunctional medicines system. "That is amazing," Lyon thought. Then she thought some more. "*I* could do that."

So, on World Cancer Day in 2016, Lyon joined Heckscher in a sit-in at the Washington, DC, headquarters of the Pharmaceutical Researchers and Manufacturers Association (PhRMA). The organization is a coalition of pharmaceutical corporations that spends billions of dollars in political lobbying and campaign contributions, all to protect medicine patent monopolies—and the record-setting profits those monopolies provide. Wearing matching black t-shirts with white lettering that read, "I am a cancer patient. No TPP death sentence," Lyon and Heckscher blocked the building entrance. "We will not leave until PhRMA stops pushing extreme monopolies through the Trans-Pacific Partnership," they said.

Outside, demonstrators from a World Cancer Day action coordinated by the advocacy group Public Citizen could see Lyon and Heckscher lock arms. The crowd got excited and increased the volume on its chants: "Shame on PhRMA!" "TPP no!" By now, someone was filming, so Lyon and Heckscher looked at the camera. "We have a message for Congress on World Cancer Day. Listen to the cancer patients who will suffer if the TPP is approved."[2] They were arrested and charged with unlawful entry.

Soon after, Lyon and Heckscher formed a new organization, Cancer Families for Affordable Medicine (CancerFAM).[3] CancerFAM is devoted, first, to stopping the TPP and, then, to fixing the other pharma-pushed trade deals and laws that elevate profits over patients. Lyon says advocacy has empowered her and transformed her own cancer story from one of weakness to one of strength. She believes that others can follow the same path.

Sarah Jackson does not have cancer, but she faces the same challenge that many of Hannah Lyon's fellow cancer patients do. The mother of six children, Sarah Jackson has hepatitis C (hep C), a blood-borne virus that can inflame and scar the liver, damaging its ability to filter toxins. Sometimes hep C causes cancer and liver failure. Sarah Jackson's physician has prescribed her a medicine to treat her disease. The medicine is almost certain to cure her before the hepatitis virus can cause irreparable liver damage or trigger liver cancer. The medicine would also prevent her from spreading the virus to others, including any future children she may give birth to.[4]

Sarah Jackson does not live in an impoverished country. She lives in Fort Wayne, Indiana, in the United States, one of the wealthiest countries in the world and the country that spends far and away the most on health care.[5] Nevertheless, Sarah Jackson cannot get access to the medicine she needs.

The medicine that Sarah Jackson's physician has prescribed her is sofosbuvir, a new hepatitis C drug that is controlled under patent by the U.S.-based pharmaceutical company Gilead. Gilead markets sofosbuvir under the names Sovaldi and Harvoni. The company has taken advantage of its monopoly patent power to price Sovaldi and Harvoni at costs that approach $1,000 per pill. The recommended twelve-week regimen cost as much as $100,000.[6]

That price is so forbidding that U.S. private insurance companies and the U.S. Veterans Administration have refused to approve the use of the drug for some patients, even when clinical treatment guidelines called for it.[7] A 2015 study published in the journal *Annals of Internal Medicine* showed that three-quarters of state Medicaid programs block many patients from receiving sofosbuvir despite their doctor's insisting they need it.[8] A U.S.

Senate investigation concluded that only about 2 percent of Medicaid patients with hepatitis C were being treated with sofosbuvir.[9] And the problem is not limited to the United States. A World Health Organization study showed the price of the drug exceeded annual per capita income levels in many countries with high hepatitis C infection rates. For example, in Poland, Portugal, Slovakia, and Turkey, a course of sofosbuvir costs at least two years of average annual wages.[10]

One of the U.S. state programs that rations the use of sofosbuvir is in Indiana, where Sarah Jackson is enrolled in Medicaid. Indiana officials refuse to pay for the medicine for hepatitis C patients until the patients' disease has progressed to the point of causing advanced liver damage. Sarah Jackson has not endured that much damage yet, so her doctor's application to have the medicine provided was denied. The doctor appealed to higher-ups in the program, but to no avail.

Then the doctor put Jackson in touch with public interest lawyers. With the lawyers' help, she has filed suit on behalf of thousands of others in Indiana who were in the same situation, asking for Medicaid to provide the medicine when their physicians say they need it. Sarah Jackson had never intended to become an activist. But, like Hannah Lyon, her illness pushed her in that direction. "There's nowhere else to go," she says. "The doctor tried and now I have no other place to turn."[11]

Rationing plans such as the one in Indiana have angered patient advocacy groups and veterans' organizations, and they have caused a passionate but less public backlash from treating physicians.[12] On the other side, the administrators of the government health care systems are in a tight spot. The state of Kentucky spent 7 percent of its total 2014 Medicaid budget, over $50 million, solely on Gilead drugs to treat just 861 hepatitis C patients.[13] The Veterans Administration was reported to have spent $1 billion on the drugs in the 2016 fiscal year.[14] When a reporter asked him to comment on Sarah Jackson's situation, Matt Salo, director of the National Association of Medicaid Directors said, "With the price of hepatitis C drugs, it is just not feasible to provide it to everyone."[15]

As that comment suggests, Sarah Jackson is far from alone. An estimated 2.7 million people in the United States are infected with hepatitis C, and its complications cause 15,000 U.S. deaths each year.[16] Globally, 150 million are infected and a half-million die from hepatitis C–related causes annually.[17] The World Health Organization calls the disease a "viral time bomb."[18] In the United States, a recent spike in intravenous drug use, chiefly among young people, has triggered a corresponding burst of new hepatitis C infections.[19] The rate of infection among U.S. military veterans is significantly higher than in the general population, partly due to exposure to blood in combat and training and to transfusions conducted before routine blood screenings began in 1992. According to the Veterans Administration, more than 200,000 U.S. military veterans are likely to have hepatitis C.[20]

The good news for those diagnosed with hepatitis C is that sofosbuvir is a remarkably effective treatment, combining with other drugs to cure the infection in more than 90 percent of patients.[21] The bad news is that Gilead has responded to the high demand for this wonder drug by setting a take-it-or-leave-it price that is 1,000 times greater than the company's manufacturing costs.[22] Advocates and even some government agencies have leveled accusations of price gouging, pointing out that the cost of a full regimen of sofosbuvir in Egypt and India is just $900, a 99 percent reduction from the U.S. price.[23] The Nobel Peace Prize–winning health care and advocacy organization Médecins Sans Frontières/Doctors Without Borders (MSF), estimates that the probable generic cost of the drug regimen would be under $200, or about 1/500 of the price currently charged to U.S. patients.[24]

The response by Gilead to its critics is the boilerplate argument from patent-holding pharmaceutical corporations: high drug prices are necessary to support research and development efforts.[25] But it turns out that government funding was the critical component in the development of sofosbuvir, not corporate investment.[26] As we see in chapter 14, this is a common phenomenon in drug research, with major advancements reliably supported by the same taxpayers who are later required to pay high prices set by corporations that possess government-granted patent monopolies.[27] In the business of medicines, the new product risks are socialized, but profits are privatized.

2

THE UNITED STATES
HAS A DRUG PROBLEM

The corporation Gilead owns the patent on sofosbuvir, the medicine that Sarah Jackson and millions of others with hepatitis C need. That patent awards the corporation a monopoly that allows it to set the price of sofosbuvir at whatever level the corporation believes the market will bear. Gilead has bet that the market will bear an astronomical price for a desperately needed medicine, and that bet has paid off, particularly in the United States, where aggressive pharmaceutical industry lobbying has blocked overall price regulation and even the ability of the government to negotiate the prices of the drugs it purchases itself.[1] Gilead collected $12 billion in hepatitis C drug sales revenue in 2014, at least half of it paid by U.S. government agencies.[2] That kind of income allows the company to pay John Martin, its CEO, as much as $180 million per year.[3]

The crisis caused by monopoly drug pricing is not limited to hepatitis C patients such as Sarah Jackson.[4] There are many other examples of essential medicines being priced out of the reach of patients in the United States and in other wealthy nations. For example, spending on medicine for diabetes, a disease diagnosed in 29 million Americans, is higher per patient than any other traditional drug class, in part because more than half of diabetes prescriptions filled are for patented drugs.[5] The cost for insulin lispro, marketed by the pharmaceutical corporation Eli Lilly under the name Humalog, increased by 325 percent from 2010 to 2015.[6] There were only two other insulin manufacturers in the United States, Sanofi and Novo Nordisk, and they also hiked their prices over 100 percent in that time span. There is no generic form of insulin, and the lack of price regulation of medicines in the United States keeps prices up to six times higher than in other developed nations, a situation that U.S. Senator Jon Tester (D-MT) labeled "price gouging, plain and simple."[7]

Not surprisingly, U.S. physicians report routinely seeing patients whose lives are at risk because they cannot afford to use the prescribed amount of insulin.[8] A 2017 lawsuit alleging price collusion among the insulin manufacturers includes reports of U.S. patients injecting expired insulin, starving themselves to control their blood sugars, and intentionally allowing themselves to slip into dangerous states of diabetic ketoacidosis so they could get free insulin samples from hospital emergency rooms.[9] In low-income countries, the situation is even more dire. A diabetes patient advocate reported a 2017 conversation with a physician in Cameroon, who shared the story of a young patient's father happily delivering news. "Did you hear? Isabelle died!" the father said with a smile. He was referring to his diabetic daughter (the name here is a pseudonym), whose need for insulin and equipment like syringes and blood sugar test strips had plunged the family into financial distress. "Now we are all able to eat enough, and the other children can get an education."[10]

In addition to insulin, similarly high costs are faced by U.S. patients in need of medicine to address heart disease, high cholesterol, and infections.[11] Vaccines are priced so high that one-third of U.S. family physicians say they are considering ending their practice of offering vaccinations because they cannot afford to buy them and keep them in stock.[12] In 2015, Turing Pharmaceuticals suddenly increased by 5,000 percent the price of its anti-infection drug Daraprim. Overnight, the price rose from $13.50 to $750.00 per tablet, a spike that brought the annual cost of treatment to as much as a half million dollars.[13] From 2007 to 2016, Mylan Pharmaceuticals hiked the price of the lifesaving anti-allergy medicine EpiPen by nearly 500 percent.[14] Although the audacity of these price hikes generated instant outrage—the two 2016 major-party U.S. presidential candidates called the Daraprim spike "price gouging" (Hillary Clinton) and "disgusting" (Donald Trump)—they were just extreme examples of the common industry practice.[15] From 2012 to 2015, list prices on medicines made by large pharmaceutical corporations rose by over 12 percent per year, far exceeding the less than 2 percent annual rate of inflation over that period and also far exceeding the increase in other health care costs.[16] In 2015, drug prices in the United States rose by almost 16 percent.[17]

Those rising prices are a predictable result of the U.S. approach to medicines, which includes a unique combination of huge government spending on medicines paired with no regulation of medicine prices (a combination I explore more fully in chapter 15).[18] The result is an environment with no price restraints. "Medicare is a huge, guaranteed market," one industry observer says. "So the (pharmaceutical) companies are saying, 'Let 'er rip!'"[19]

So it is not surprising that U.S. patients pay the highest prices for medicine in the world, a per capita cost of about $1,000 per year.[20] Consider this:

- A recent study showed that the median monthly price of branded cancer drugs in the United States was almost $8,700, compared with about $2,600 in the United Kingdom, $2,700 in Australia, and $3,200 in China.[21]
- In the United States, medicines represent 10 percent of national spending on health and nearly 20 percent of spending in employer health insurance plans.[22]
- Overall prescription drug spending in the United States is over $400 billion annually; global spending exceeds $1 trillion.[23] Some European health systems, which unlike the U.S. Medicare program do negotiate drug prices, have even refused to pay for some high-cost medicines.[24]

Ultimately, these whopping U.S. medicine bills are paid by the taxpayers who subsidize government health care programs such as Medicare and Medicaid. They are also paid by private health care systems, whose CEOs' report that rising drug costs are undermining the finances of their companies.[25] Increasingly, the costs incurred by those private companies are passed on to patients. Even when U.S. residents are covered by private insurance plans, those plans usually charge premiums and copayments, and do not cover costs until a deductible threshold is met. In the last decade, U.S. workers' obligations for those health insurance premiums rose 83 percent and their deductibles rose 255 percent, with 2016 testimony to a U.S. Senate committee identifying prescription drug prices as the biggest reason for those increases.[26] One of the results of this crisis is that medical debt has become the single largest cause of bankruptcy in the United States.[27]

As Sarah Jackson can attest, for many patients, the high cost of medicines simply means that a doctor's prescription goes unfilled. In a 2015 U.S. poll, 19 percent of respondents said they had recently not filled a prescription because they could not afford the price.[28] Another survey reported that 50 million Americans each year skip taking prescribed medication due to the cost.[29] Predictably, there is a human price to be paid for missing medications: multiple studies have shown that persons who struggle to access prescribed drugs are at greater risk of heart attacks, strokes, and other life-threatening health emergencies.[30]

Even when patients do have adequate insurance coverage or can afford to pay out of pocket the cost of the medicine they need, they often discover that the medicine is still not available to them. In the United States, medicine shortages are reported to be "the new normal," with regular gaps in the availability of essential antibiotics, cancer drugs, and anesthetics, among hundreds of other medicines.[31] In 2013, 83 percent of U.S. cancer physicians reported not being able to provide a patient with the preferred chemotherapy at least once in the previous six months. One-third of those physicians reported having to delay treatment or exclude patients from the medicine altogether.[32] Reports of medicine rationing have been registered in the treatment of leukemia, ovarian cancer, bladder cancer, and infections in need of antibiotics.[33] Some U.S. physicians admit they deliberately avoid telling their patients that they are not getting the medicine they need.[34]

Like high prices, these shortages are the inevitable consequence of a medicine system built on a foundation that relies on the motivations of corporations seeking the highest possible profits. If pharmaceutical corporations determine there is not sufficient money to be made producing a medicine, especially compared to other products that they can charge enormous mark-ups for, they have no incentive to make enough of the medicines that have lower profit margins. The shortages are also spurred on by the secretive, exclusive character of the patent system, which leads to a limited number of manufacturers of the needed drugs.[35]

Even if the medicines that are in shortage are potentially profitable to manufacture, "intellectual property" rights often trump patient needs. For example, when the Cleveland Clinic responded to a shortage of a blood-vessel surgery drug by mixing up its own version in-house, the clinic physicians wanted to share the formula with their colleagues facing similar shortages in other hospitals. But they discovered they could not do so: the Cleveland Clinic had claimed exclusive rights to the combination.[36]

Sometimes drug shortages are the result of quality control issues in the medicine manufacturing process. But that problem too can be traced back to the for-profit nature of the industry because corporations see little urgency in fixing the manufacturing problem for a medicine that produces limited revenue. As a journalist who investigated drug shortages said, "Sometimes what happens is a [production] line goes down, something breaks down and a company, a producer looks at the margins and the economics and says 'well, you know it's not really worth the margins we're getting on this drug in continuing the line—in putting the money in to fix it.' So they let the drug go into shortage. And even if people need it—say it's nitroglycerine which is critical in heart surgery—they just don't produce it."[37]

Instead, for-profit pharmaceutical corporations inevitably focus their investments and their production capacity on medicines that provide a hefty profit. We have already read about one example: the hepatitis C medicine with a 500 percent mark-up (chapter 1). Not surprisingly, there have been no reported shortages of Sovaldi or Harvoni.

3

MILLIONS OF PEOPLE
ARE DYING NEEDLESSLY

Tobeka Daki lived with her two sons in the Mdanstane Township in the Eastern Cape province of South Africa. Her youngest son, Khanya, is eleven years old. She was a breast cancer patient, struggling with a particularly aggressive strain of the disease known as HER2.[1]

Trastuzumab is a medicine that is effective in treating HER2-positive breast cancer.[2] Marketed under the brand name Herceptin by the pharmaceutical company Roche, the medicine is so successful at improving survival rates for HER2 patients such as Tobeka that the World Health Organization has placed it on its "Essential Medicines List," an exclusive category of drugs that are considered necessary to meet the minimum medicine needs for a basic health care system.[3] The development of trastuzumab was so impactful that the story was turned into a Lifetime TV movie, *Living Proof*, starring Harry Connick Jr. as the physician whose research helped show that the medicine would benefit cancer patients. Herceptin has become one of the best-selling prescription drugs in the world.[4]

The cost to manufacture a year's worth of trastuzumab, the recommended length of treatment for a patient such as Tobeka, is about $176.[5] Yet that same amount of medicine is sold by Roche in South Africa at a price of about $34,000.[6] The company holds the South African patent for the medicine until 2033; this means that there are no competitors to push Roche to lower the price. Roche sells over $6 billion of the medicine each year.[7]

The $34,000 price tag for trastuzumab was far more than Tobeka could pay. The same goes for the vast majority of other HER2-positive breast cancer patients in South Africa, where the per capita income is $6,800.[8] Few private insurers cover the drug. The public-sector health care system so rarely provides trastuzumab that physicians in that system usually do not even tell their HER2 patients about the existence of the drug.[9]

When I spoke with Tobeka in March 2016, she explained that her cancer had recently spread to her spine, so she had officially reached the Stage 4 level. Her sons were distraught. One of her fellow patients, with whom she had grown close, had died five days before. "Thousands of people in South Africa die because they cannot access this medicine," she said.[10] Tobeka Daki died in November, 2016. She never received trastuzumab.[11]

The story of Tobeka, Roche, and trastuzumab is just one version of a story that can be repeated for millions of patients and hundreds of lifesaving medicines across the world. The fact that this particular story is set in South Africa is sadly ironic. South Africa was the center of the historic struggle to dramatically increase access to HIV/AIDS drugs, a struggle described in the conclusion of this book. By challenging patent medicine monopolies, South African activists won a victory that ensures that millions of Tobeka's countrymen and countrywomen receive affordable antiretroviral therapy for HIV/AIDS.

But trastuzumab and many other medicines remain protected by patents and priced out of reach. Some say that means that medicine activists won the HIV/AIDS treatment battle but have lost the broader access-to-medicine war. But others say the victory won for HIV/AIDS medicines is possible for other kinds of drugs, too. Lillian Dube, also a South African woman with breast cancer, was struck by the sight of her fellow patients, such as Tobeka, going without the medicine they need. "I am with young women (at our doctor). These are women who are 40, 30, and they have small children," Dube says. "And they have to lose their lives because they cannot afford Herceptin. It should not be like that."[12]

As I show in this book, there are dozens of reasons why Lillian Dube is right: it should not be like that. And there are many activists such as Lillian Dube who are working to change the system. "Until I die, I'll be fighting this," she says.[13]

Ahmed is a little boy, and he is dying. He could be in India or Nigeria or Haiti. And he could be dying from pneumonia or diarrhea or measles.

Unlike Tobeka Daki, Ahmed is not one particular person. He cannot tell his story to an interviewer. He lays anonymous, engulfed in fever, in a hut in a remote village or in a shack in a teeming urban slum. Neither his family nor his government could afford to give him the immunizations that would have prevented his illness. And they cannot afford the antibiotic medicines that would help him survive now.

One out of every five children living in poor countries never receives even the most basic package of vaccinations.[14] Millions do not have access to antibiotic drugs.[15] Ahmed is one of 6 million children in low- and middle-income countries who will die from an infectious disease this year.[16] Chances are that his disease is pneumonia because that is the leading cause of childhood death, in large part because three out of four of the world's children have not been vaccinated against it.[17]

There are massive global efforts to expand the vaccination of children, such as Ahmed. Gavi, the Vaccine Alliance, leverages funding from the Bill and Melinda Gates Foundation and from other public and private sources, to immunize millions of children in low-income countries.[18] MSF delivers nearly 7 million doses of vaccines each year.[19] But even these efforts were not enough to reach Ahmed, and they will not reach millions of other children.

The biggest reason is the cost of the medicines. Dr. Greg Elder, deputy director of operations for Médecins Sans Frontières, says, "The rising price of the basic vaccines package means that we can't afford to protect kids living in crisis."[20] That price for a full package of vaccines in 2014 was sixty-eight times what it was in 2001.[21] The most expensive vaccine in that package is the pneumococcal vaccine, which generates almost $7 billion in sales each year for the pharmaceutical corporations GSK and Pfizer, which control the market for the drug.[22] In late 2016, a determined multiyear advocacy campaign led by MSF finally succeeded in convincing the two chief producers of the pneumococcal vaccine to lower the prices they charged humanitarian organizations. But advocates cautioned that, even after the price drop, the vaccine was still unaffordable in many poor countries.[23]

Tobeka and Ahmed are not isolated examples. The UN World Health Organization says that one-third of the world's population do not have access to essential medicines.[24] Other UN health officials estimate that 10 million people die each year because they do not receive the medicines that would have saved them.[25] That adds up to one person dying every three seconds—more people each year than the entire population of New York City.

The World Health Organization and others can categorize that number by the diseases that are left unchecked. Over a million die each year from tuberculosis, and a million-plus more from AIDS, malaria, and hepatitis.[26] Those dying from infectious diseases such as these tend to be younger, like Ahmed. But millions more, like Tobeka, die prematurely from untreated noncommunicable diseases such as cancer, cardiovascular disease, and diabetes.[27]

The 2015 annual report of the World Health Organization sounds like a broken record repeating the same tragic notes:

- Access to medicines for noncommunicable diseases "is still very poor in many low- and lower-middle income countries."[28]
- A majority of newborns who need hepatitis B immunizations do not get them, and most cancer patients who need chemotherapy do not get that either.[29]
- New cancer and hepatitis medicines are enormously effective, but as we have learned (chapters 1 and 2), they are "largely unaffordable while under patent, even for many high-income countries."[30]
- For diabetes patients in low-income countries, "essential medicines are frequently unavailable or unaffordable."[31] Same goes for patients in need of mental health medicines.[32]

Even when the lack of medicines is not immediately fatal, it often makes survival a miserable experience: billions of people lack access to opioid analgesics that can ease the excruciating pain of diseases such as cancer.[33] Those lucky enough to be able to buy essential medicines often make enormous sacrifices to do so. As much as 90 percent of people in low- and middle-income countries pay out of pocket for their medicines, making it the second-largest family expenditure after food.[34] In these countries, medicine costs account for nearly half of all health care spending, drawing resources away from hiring doctors and nurses, building clinics, and buying other supplies.[35]

This crisis has not gone unnoticed. Thomas Pogge, a Yale University philosopher, calls this poverty-induced suffering and death "the morally pre-eminent problem of our age."[36] The global community has recently agreed on a set of Sustainable Development Goals that includes achieving universal access to essential medicines.[37] In 2015, the UN secretary-general convened a High-Level Panel on Access to Medicines, emphasizing the urgency of the situation, and the panel issued a report underscoring that millions are dying of treatable diseases because they cannot access needed medicines.[38]

But the suffering of Tobeka, Ahmed, and millions of others continues. There is no more stark example of our broken medicines system than the Ebola epidemic of 2014.

On October 13, 2014, Dr. Margaret Chan, the director-general of the World Health Organization, provided the keynote address for the sixty-fifth session of the WHO Regional Committee for the Western Pacific.[39] Most conferences like this are highly bureaucratic; the speeches delivered are typically long on platitudes and short on drama. But Dr. Chan's remarks were delivered in the midst of the Ebola outbreak in western Africa, an outbreak she told the attendees had generated more fear than any event in her public health career.

So Dr. Chan took the occasion, and the global media attention to the outbreak, as an opportunity to be remarkably frank. Over 11,000 people will die from Ebola, she said. "The outbreak spotlights the dangers of the world's growing social and economic inequalities," she told the attendees. "The rich get the best care. The poor are left to die."[40]

Dr. Chan was correct. Ebola was a dramatic example of the inequities in the global health care system, inequities that are particularly stark in the field of medicines. The reason Ebola was so frightening and so deadly was that no medicines were available to prevent it or to treat it. It turns out that promising vaccines to prevent Ebola, and drugs to treat it, had been uncovered years before the outbreak. Yet they were allowed to languish without further development. "There is a lesson here," said

Professor Adrian Hill from Oxford University, who led the Ebola response for Britain. "If we had invested in an Ebola vaccine, had it sitting there as the outbreak comes, you could have nipped it in the bud, been able to vaccinate the region when it started."[41]

So why was the Ebola vaccine not developed? Because pharmaceutical corporations saw no prospect of significant profit to be made on the drug. The expected need was limited, and those who would benefit were likely to be too poor to pay high prices. As far back as 2003, Thomas Geisbert, an Ebola researcher, recognized the problem, writing with regret that there was "little commercial interest for developing an Ebola virus vaccine."[42]

After the 2014 outbreak began claiming lives by the thousands, Professor Hill labeled the problem in stark terms. "Who makes vaccines? Today, commercial vaccine supply is monopolized by four or five mega-companies—GSK, Sanofi, Merck, Pfizer—some of the biggest companies in the world," Hill said. "The problem with that it, even if you've got a way of making the vaccine, unless there's a big market, it's not worth the while of a mega-company. . . . There was no business case to make an Ebola vaccine for the people who needed it the most."[43]

The 11,000 people who died from Ebola are just the latest and most visible examples of a core flaw of the for-profit medicine system. Medicines that address the diseases that kill millions of the global poor do not present a compelling business case. The U.S. satirical publication *The Onion* put a sadly accurate spin on the tragic situation, publishing a spoof article entitled "Experts: Ebola Vaccine at Least 50 White People Away,"[44]

So medicines that would save the lives of the global poor go undeveloped. All the while, for-profit corporations rush to market hair-loss cures and erectile dysfunction drugs. Such medicines often duplicate others on the market and are often frivolous compared to other needed medicines. But they still present a good business case, as long as they address the real or perceived needs of consumers who can pay high prices.

As she concluded her October 2014 speech, Dr. Chan did not shy away from identifying the obvious cause for the 11,000 deaths. "Ebola emerged 40 years ago. Why are clinicians still empty-handed, with no vaccines and no cure? Because Ebola has been, historically, geographically confined to poor African nations.

"The R&D [research and development] incentive is virtually non-existent. A profit-driven industry does not invest in products for markets that cannot pay."[45]

4

CANCER PATIENTS FACE PARTICULARLY
DEADLY BARRIERS TO MEDICINES

In 2013, I was diagnosed with testicular seminoma. Fortunately for me, this is a form of cancer that is highly treatable. Even more fortunate for me, I could access that treatment. I live in an area where top-level care is available, I had good insurance coverage through my employer, and I could afford to pay out-of-pocket costs. I am now healthy and have every reason to believe the cancer is gone.

Some of you may have had your own experiences of cancer, either as a patient yourself or as a friend or family member of someone who has had cancer. There are 14 million new cases of cancer diagnosed annually.[1]

If you or a loved one has faced cancer, you already know about the breathtaking cost of the medicines used in its treatment. In 2012, the U.S. Food and Drug Administration (FDA) approved twelve new cancer drugs. Eleven of them were priced over $100,000 per year per patient.[2] One drug used to treat acute lymphoblastic leukemia, patented by the company Amgen, costs $178,000 for the standard course of treatment.[3] Over the past decade, cancer treatment costs have increased 39 percent in inflation-adjusted terms.[4] The average price for a patented cancer drug in the United States now exceeds $10,000 per month, and the global market for oncology medicines is over $100 billion per year.[5] Even for a U.S. patient with health insurance, typical out-of-pocket costs of 20–30 percent leave the patient paying $20,000–$30,000 annually for cancer medicines, an amount equal to about half the average U.S. household's income.[6]

The driving force behind these astronomical prices is neither manufacturing costs nor investments in research and development. Cancer drugs cost so much because monopoly-protected patented medicines are priced at whatever the market will bear. And the market will bear enormous prices when patients and their families are desperate to save or prolong lives.

A peek inside the pricing system proves the point. In December 2015, the *Wall Street Journal* published an inside account of how Pfizer executives decided to set the price of a new breast cancer drug. The corporate calculations were focused on discovering the maximum price that insurers would be willing to pay and the price level at which physicians would balk at prescribing the drug. Worried about the intimidating nature of a price of $10,000 per month, the Pfizer team tapped into the same tactics of misdirection that cause microwave ovens and flat-screen TVs to so often carry price tags ending with $99 or 99 cents. Pfizer decided that the new breast cancer drug would be sold at $9,850 per month.[7] "At some point, it's just corporate chutzpah," Dr. Peter Bach of the Memorial Sloan-Kettering Cancer Center says of the cancer drug–pricing process in general. "There's no check on the system."[8]

But what if there were checks on the system and cancer medicines were priced at a level that reflected their costs of production plus a reasonable profit for the manufacturer? How much would these medicines cost then? In 2015, a team of British and U.S. researchers set out to make that price calculation for four potent cancer medicines. The medicines examined were all in a category called tyrosine kinase inhibitors: imatinib, used to treat leukemia; erlotinib, used to treat lung and pancreatic cancer; lapatinib, used to treat breast cancer; and sorafenib, used to treat kidney and liver cancer. The researchers tallied up the costs of production and packaging for all these medicines and added in a generous 50 percent profit margin. Remarkably, the total prices determined by this process were less than 10 percent of the current patent-protected prices. For one of the medicines, imatinib, the researcher's estimated price was less than 1/600 of the current price.[9]

The difference between the actual costs of cancer medicines and the monopoly patent mark-up is measurable, not just in dollars—the gap in pricing means that lives are lost as well. We have already read (chapter 3) how Tobeka Daki's survival depends on a breast cancer medicine she cannot afford. Millions of others face the same barrier: while the cancer fatality rate is 46.4 percent in high-income countries, the rate is 74.5 percent in low-income countries.[10] The cancer treatment challenges of the global poor extend beyond medicines, of course. There is a lack of robust health care systems providing opportunities for early detection and nonpharmaceutical treatment such as radiation.[11] Sometimes those challenges are cited by the pharmaceutical companies as a justification for their high prices. In 2016, the CEO of AstraZeneca, Pascal Soriot, claimed that, "In some parts of Africa, we could give our products away and it would make no difference."[12]

But the health care systems are improving in many areas, and the availability of medicines has not kept pace. Effective new treatments for cancer that are saving lives in wealthier countries are not available to the global poor due to their price, regardless of whether robust systems of care are in place. Patients in just six countries—the United States, Germany, the United Kingdom, Italy, France, and Canada—have access to more than half the oncology drugs that have been rolled out in the last five years.[13] Even when the medicine is available and a care system is in place, patients in poorer countries often cannot pay. In Nigeria, for example, a reported 63 percent of cancer patients cannot keep up with the prescribed chemotherapy due to the price of the medicines.[14]

Such precise numbers are not available everywhere. With so many poor people across the world suffering from untreated cancer in painful anonymity, researchers have struggled to make a solid estimate of the number of deaths that could have been prevented. Yet one 2010 study of available cancer treatments in poor countries concludes, in regard to those deaths, "Available information suggests that the number is probably staggering."[15] With the incidence of cancer on the rise, many global health experts hear the echoes of the 1990s HIV/AIDS crisis in the tragedy of these preventable deaths; once again, the medicines to save lives exist and can be cheaply made, but monopoly patent protection is condemning millions to an early grave.[16]

Even in the wealthy United States, up to 20 percent of cancer patients do not take the medicines prescribed to them because they cannot afford them.[17] As a 2016 *Newsweek* headline put it, "Many Cancer Patients Must Face Bankruptcy or Die."[18] This state of affairs has angered U.S. cancer physicians, including my own doctor.

In the mid-1970s, testicular cancer that had spread beyond the abdomen was considered a terminal diagnosis. Then, Lawrence Einhorn, a Indiana University School of Medicine professor and oncologist, developed a revolutionary multidrug approach that transformed the disease into a cancer that had a higher cure rate than any other.[19] More than three decades later, when I was fortunate enough to have Dr. Einhorn treating me, I found him to be deeply frustrated by the cost of medicines for his patients. In August 2015, Einhorn and 117 other leading U.S. cancer experts co-authored a commentary in the journal *Mayo Clinic Proceedings*. They pointed out that drug companies have been hiking the cost of cancer medicines by leaps and bounds, far exceeding the rate of inflation. "This raises the question of whether current pricing of cancer drugs is based on reasonable expectation of return on investment or whether it is based on what prices the market can bear," the oncologists wrote.[20]

In their article, Einhorn and his fellow oncologists call for the U.S. Medicare program to be allowed to negotiate the price of drugs and for limits on patent-holders' delaying the availability of generic alternatives. (We learn more about these ideas in chapters 20 and 21.) And they urge cancer patients to follow the lead of HIV/AIDS patients, whose political advocacy in the 1990s and early 2000s led to a sharp decrease in drug prices.[21] "There is no question that you need an incentive to develop new medicines," Einhorn told me. "But, in terms of cost, how much is too much? You have families facing bankruptcy due to the cost of healthcare, and medicines are a part of that problem."[22]

The lead author of the article, Ayalew Tefferi, a hematologist at Mayo Clinic, was more blunt. After the publication of the article, he told the *Wall Street Journal,* "What we're fighting is the greed."[23] Drs. Einhorn and Tefferi and their colleagues were following in the footsteps of experts in chronic myeloid leukemia (CML), who wrote in their professional journal *Blood* in 2013, "As physicians, we follow the Hippocratic Oath of 'Primum non nocere,' first (or above all) do no harm. We believe the unsustainable drug prices in CML and cancer may be causing harm to patients. Advocating for lower drug prices is a necessity to save the lives of patients who cannot afford them."[24]

In 2016, cancer physicians reported a new reason for anger at pharmaceutical corporations. Researchers from the New York City Memorial Sloan Kettering Cancer Center published a study in *BMJ* (formerly known as the *British Medical Journal*), reporting that as much as $3 billion was being spent each year by Medicare and private insurers—and patients who were making copayments—for chemotherapy drugs that had to be thrown away.[25] The medicine is purchased but wasted because the manufacturers intentionally sell it in vials that contain a dose that is far too large for the average person.

An example provided by the study is the medicine Velcade, sold by Takeda Pharmaceuticals for the treatment of multiple myeloma and lymphoma, and available in the United States only in vials that contain enough medicine to treat a person who is 6 feet, 6 inches tall and who weighs 250 pounds. For anyone smaller, the dose is less and much of that medicine is not used. Safety rules mandate that leftover medicine must be discarded—even though the drug company has charged for the larger amount. "Drug companies are quietly making billions forcing little old ladies to buy enough medicine to treat football players," said one of the researchers.[26]

Although cancer physicians are increasingly upset about medicine pricing, few cancer patient groups have challenged the drug patent status quo. That seems puzzling at first, given that many patient advocacy groups are well-funded, well-known in policy circles, and usually quite vocal about treatment and research issues. As it turns out, however, many of these groups rely on the pharmaceutical industry for organizational funding and sometimes for donations of unaffordable medicines to desperate patients.[27] A September 2016 *New York Times* article noted that patient advocacy groups were "oddly muted" in the EpiPen and "Pharma Bro"–fueled high-profile drug-pricing debates. Perhaps the silence is not so odd after all: the same article chronicled how the National Multiple Sclerosis Society endured pushback from its pharma funders when it dared to mention concerns over the price of multiple sclerosis drugs averaging $78,000 annually, a 400 percent increase in little over a decade.[28]

Moreover, quite often pharma-funded patient advocacy groups break their silence on drug-pricing debates to affirmatively side with industry resistance to reform. A 2016 Public Citizen report revealed that at least three-quarters of the patient groups that actively opposed an Obama administration proposal to reduce Medicare drug expenditures had received pharma-industry donations; another study showed that over 90 percent of patient groups participating in a discussion of FDA drug approval reform were pharma-funded.[29] Most patient groups that opposed the 2016 California Proposition 61 ballot measure to regulate the medicine prices paid by the state government had received significant financial support from the pharmaceutical corporations.[30]

It is no wonder that those corporations enlist patient advocacy groups to make their case: the groups provide the moral authority and individual stories that can sway undecided lawmakers and voters. For example, one response to a 2016 blog post in *HealthNewsReview* that discussed industry funding of patient advocacy groups was "Until you have been a patient, you don't know what it is like. . . . Pharma and biotech are developing science that literally saves the lives of people like me."[31] The power of such testimonials is undeniable, and the honesty of the patients who speak out should not be questioned. Nevertheless, their arguments are indelibly tainted when they are sponsored by corporate money. As one researcher wrote in the *BMJ*, "A consumer group funded by telephone companies would not be trusted to judge the best mobile phone package, nor to be a public advocate on telecommunications policy. Is health less important?"[32]

But, as we have seen in the story of Hannah Lyon and Zahara Heckscher (chapter 1), cancer patients and cancer groups are becoming more outspoken about medicine prices. As I discuss in the conclusion of this book, patient advocacy groups played critical roles in HIV/AIDS and other treatment campaigns. They may end up playing a similarly impactful role in cancer treatment, too. Take the example of South African cancer survivor and activist Linda Greeff, founder of the group People Living with Cancer, who was moved by the stories of untreated South African cancer patients such as Tobeka Daki. After Greef turned her attention to patent law reform efforts, her group quickly lost some of its pharmaceutical corporate funding. But Greeff says she is willing to accept the trade-off. She has been able to hang on to a few industry donations, and she makes clear that she accepts them with no strings attached. "I tell them we will take your money, but we will not be singing your song!" she says.[33]

5

THE CURRENT MEDICINE SYSTEM
NEGLECTS MANY MAJOR DISEASES

As we have seen in chapter 3, thousands of people died from Ebola because our current medicines system ignored the health needs of the low-income patients who faced the risk of that epidemic. The Ebola tragedy is just one indicator of the flaw lying at the heart of our medicine development process. For pharmaceutical corporations, the pot at the end of the research rainbow is filled with gold only if the discovered medicine can be sold at high prices to patients or their government health care systems.

Inevitably, this arrangement means that pharmaceutical corporations devote their research almost exclusively to medicines that will be consumed by the comparatively wealthy. Researchers Adam Mannan and Alan Story have pointed out that the corporate marketing dollars spent to promote any one of the current high-profile erectile dysfunction drugs far exceed the global investment in developing a vaccine for dengue fever, which poses a risk to 40 percent of the world's population.[1] And little wonder, given the for-profit foundation of the current system: within a day of the introduction of the erectile dysfunction drug Viagra, the stock price of Pfizer, its patent-holder, doubled.[2]

In global health discussions, the term used for killers such as dengue fever, along with elephantiasis, sleeping sickness, river blindness, and others, is *neglected diseases*. These diseases have a ferocious impact: one of every six people in the world, including a half billion children, suffer from neglected diseases.[3] And the moniker *neglected* is well deserved; these diseases represent barely a blip on the radar screen of medicine research and development. Only 4 percent of new medicines registered during the years 2000–2011 were for neglected diseases,[4] and in 2010, only about 1 percent of research and development dollars was directed at neglected diseases.[5] This is not a new phenomenon. An oft-cited analysis reported in the British medical journal *The Lancet* found that, of 1,556 new chemical entities marketed between 1975 and 2004, only 21 were for tropical diseases and tuberculosis.[6]

In contrast, pharmaceutical industry research on hair-loss treatments is going strong, and new medicines to reduce facial wrinkles and to thicken eyelashes are rushed to market. The disparity is so stark that it long ago earned its own name—the 10/90 Problem—reflecting the approximation that only 10 percent of research and development goes into creating medicines for diseases that affect 90 percent of the world's population.[7]

A particularly disturbing example of the 10/90 problem is provided by the case of tuberculosis (TB), one of the deadliest diseases in the world. More than 9 million people develop TB each year, and 1.6 million die from it annually.[8] Yet over the past half-century, only two new medicines have been developed to treat TB, and an increasing number of patients have TB that is resistant to the decades-old medicines that are the predominant form of treatment.[9] Like the Ebola vaccine, promising treatments sit undeveloped because TB mostly affects the global poor.[10]

The situation is not improving. Although there are philanthropic and government investments in TB research, major pharmaceutical corporations continue to walk away from the crisis.[11] In 2014, for example, AstraZeneca closed a major research laboratory in India devoted to TB and other neglected diseases, announcing a renewed focus on medicines for cancer, high blood pressure, and other diseases that affect people in the developed world.[12] That same year, Pfizer cancelled plans for a TB medicine clinical trial in South Africa.[13] The *Financial Times* identified these decisions as evidence of a "gloomy outlook" for privately funded research and development for TB drugs. "TB is particularly unattractive as a commercial proposition because [it] is heavily concentrated among the indigent in poorer countries," the newspaper article concluded.[14]

A similar lack of commercial appeal has stunted research for new antibiotics to respond to drug-resistant bacteria, which kill 700,000 people globally each year. In the case of drugs to address microbial resistance, the relatively short length of treatment needed has convinced for-profit pharmaceutical companies that the medicine would not be profitable.[15] Reflecting on the problems in addressing the spread of tuberculosis, antimicrobial resistance, and other health emergencies, a commission of experts empaneled by the prestigious British medical journal *The Lancet* concluded in 2016 that the present system of drug development is "in crisis."[16]

When pharmaceutical industry leaders speak candidly, they admit that all this is true. "We have no model which would meet the need for new drugs in a sustainable way," former Novartis CEO Daniel Vasella, said in 2006. "You can't expect for-profit organizations to do this in a large scale. If you want to establish a system where companies systematically invest in this kind of area [low-cost medicines for developing-countries], you need a different system."[17]

While these global health crises rage on unaddressed, the pharmaceutical industry stays laser focused on the needs of its wealthiest customers. That focus is demonstrated by a remarkable fact: nearly three of every four "new" medicines developed in recent decades are not new at all. Analyses of U.S. and French medicine development in recent decades show that over 70 percent of the medicines newly approved offer no therapeutic benefits over existing medicines.[18] Instead, the same pharmaceutical corporations that are ignoring the unprofitable diseases of the poor have devoted enormous resources to produce copycat drugs, also called "me-too" drugs, that allow them to carve out a piece of the blockbuster markets for high-end customers.[19]

One of many examples of the "me-too" phenomenon is cholesterol-reducing drugs. The United States currently has seven statins on the market to lower cholesterol, all essentially identical to the original version that was approved more than a quarter century ago.[20] Drug companies sometimes even copy themselves, creating their own version of a "me-too" drug when the patent is set to expire on the original blockbuster medicine. As the original drug is going off patent, the companies roll out a new but very similar drug and use heavy advertising to physicians and the public to move them off the older medicine, which soon will face generic competition. AstraZeneca did this, pushing the heartburn drug Nexium in place of the older Prilosec; Shering-Ploug did it, promoting Clarinex over its patent-expiring allergy drug Claritin; and Eli Lilly did it, pushing Sarafem over the antidepressant Prozac.[21]

These approaches come as no surprise. As Dr. Chan said when describing the Ebola tragedy, a medicine system based on maximizing profits creates no incentive to address the needs of the global poor, no matter how many millions of people are dying. That grim fact has been quietly acknowledged by pharmaceutical corporations for decades. On occasion, the truth is even admitted in a public setting. In a 2013 conference on the pharmaceutical industry, Marijn Dekkers, Bayer CEO, was asked about the status of one of the company cancer medicines in India. Dekkers responded with revealing candor: "We did not develop this product for the Indian market, let's be honest. We developed this product for Western patients who can afford this product, quite honestly."[22]

Part II

Profits over Patients

6

CORPORATE RESEARCH AND DEVELOPMENT INVESTMENTS ARE EXAGGERATED

We have reviewed the undeniable evidence that the pharmaceutical industry ignores the development of medicines needed by billions of people across the globe. Yet corporate spokespersons still defend the high costs of patent-protected medicines by claiming they are necessary to conduct research and development. Alan Holmer, former president of the industry trade association PhRMA, said, "Believe me, if we impose price controls on the pharmaceutical industry, and if you reduce the R&D that this industry is able to provide, it's going to harm my kids and it's going to harm those millions of other Americans who have life-threatening conditions."[1]

To buttress that argument, Holmer and his colleagues have long pointed to figures that they claim represent enormous industry expenditures for researching and developing new medicines. The most recent estimate comes from a 2014 report by the Tufts Center for the Study of Drug Development, which concluded that the average cost of bringing a drug to market is a whopping $2.6 billion.[2] That figure was quickly promoted by John J. Castellani, Holmer's successor as head of PhRMA, in newspaper articles and by his organization in colorful brochures defending existing medicine patent laws.[3]

But the accuracy of this $2.6 billion figure is highly questionable. First, consider the source: the Tufts Center reports that the institution receives 40 percent of its overall funding from the pharmaceutical industry.[4] Second, the Union for Affordable Cancer Treatment and leading medicine researchers have raised concerns about the $2.6 billion figure overstating the number of patients in and costs of the average medicine clinical trial, and the main author of the report has admitted the figure does not reflect the benefits of tax credits for the industry research, credits that could reduce corporate costs by as much as 50 percent.[5]

The questions raised about this most recent cost estimate are important because academic analyses of previous and similar reports have shown the costs to be wildly overstated. For example, Donald Light and Rebecca Warburton, health and economics researchers writing in 2011 for the London School of Economics and Political Science journal *BioSocieties*, conducted a blistering critique of a prior Tufts study of the industry research and development costs.[6] Echoing others' concerns, Light and Warburton criticized the Tufts analysis for failing to make adjustments for the substantial public investment in research and development, and for failing to identify the drugs reviewed by their therapeutic classification.[7] According to Light and Warburton, the lack of specificity in the report indicated that the cost estimates could have been conducted on a sample that was skewed toward medicines that are more expensive to develop. In fact, an unpublished appendix to the Tufts study suggested that this was indeed the case.[8]

It is similarly unclear whether the research and development estimates in the earlier Tufts study included marketing-oriented expenses, such as payments to physicians to promote the drugs or instructional courses to provide information about the drugs to prescribing physicians.[9] Light and Warburton's review suggested that half the Tufts estimate of the financial cost of research did not represent real research investments at all. Rather, it was a calculation of the income the corporations potentially would have reaped if they had not invested in research and development—a calculation that ignores the fact that those research and development costs are deducted from the taxable profits of the company each year.[10] Further, the Tufts estimate was based on clinical trials whose costs and lengths far exceeded the averages the U.S. government has reported, again suggesting the overall cost numbers were skewed upward.[11]

Not surprisingly, then, the claims by the industry for its research and development costs are widely dismissed as unreliable. Even a pharmaceutical CEO, Andrew Witty of GlaxoSmithKline, has said that the prior $1 billion estimate for developing a drug was "one of the great myths of the industry."[12] The *Economist* has labeled the current $2.6 billion figure "questionable," making special note of the padded estimates for loss of capital.[13] In addition, a coalition of academics has echoed the charge that the current Tufts estimate is "a myth."[14] Other industry observers have called into question the oft-quoted corporate estimate of thousands of compounds being tested to discover just one drug that is brought to market, noting that computerized screening of a large number of compounds is relatively quick and inexpensive.[15]

The costs to develop a medicine are variable. But, in their 2011 article, Light and Warburton concluded that the actual cost of developing a new medicine could be as low as $43.4 million, one-eighteenth of the figure the industry was promoting at the time.[16] More recent data from the nonprofit Drugs for Neglected Diseases Initiative estimate that the cost for development of a new medicine is in the range of $112 million to $169 million.[17] The Global Alliance for Tuberculosis Drug Development provides an even lower estimate for developing a new TB medicine.[18] While the industry has claimed that it costs nearly $1 billion to develop a vaccine, independent analyses put the cost at less than half that amount, and possibly as low as $150 million.[19]

Although these estimates are a fraction of the industry-promoted figures, they are still large numbers. Clinical testing of medicines is an expensive phase of the research process. Private corporations are far more eager to be involved at this stage that immediately precedes the hoped-for profits than they are in the riskier early stages, so private industry shoulders most of the clinical trials costs.[20] Nevertheless, placed in the context of a trillion-dollar industry, the costs simply do not back up the argument that the purpose of high corporate medicine profits is to support research and development investments. For example, it has been estimated that the company Novartis contributed somewhere between $38 million and $96 million to the research and development of its leukemia drug imatinib, which it markets as Gleevec. (Novartis has not disclosed its exact research and development investment, so this estimate is based on publicly available records and on past reporting of the costs of clinical trials and other research.) Novartis makes $4.7 billion in annual sales of Gleevec, which in 2016 had a wholesale U.S. cost of $120,000 per patient.[21] So, even assuming corporate costs at the highest point of the estimated range, it takes Novartis only thirteen days of Gleevec sales revenue to cover its research and development investment.[22]

More broadly, giving the pharmaceutical corporations a very generous benefit of the doubt about their actual research and development costs, and without factoring in the tax breaks associated with those costs, the industry still spends less than 15 percent of sales revenue on research and development.[23] As we see in chapter 7, the industry costs for marketing are much higher. Recent numbers reported by PhRMA suggest that the percentage of sales revenue spent on research and development is now less than 8 percent and trending downward.[24]

As they defend high medicine prices and the patents that protect them, the largest corporations still promote themselves as tireless researchers: "Our industry is poised to translate our most promising scientific breakthroughs into meaningful treatments capable of tackling the most urgent and vexing medical challenges of our times," is the quotation from Kenneth Frazier, Merck chairman and CEO, featured on PhRMA promotional material.[25] But one of the reasons for the downward trend in industry research investments is that the large pharmaceutical corporations have increasingly transitioned to a model that is less innovative and less risky than developing new drugs. The large corporations that have themselves been less successful in developing new treatments have focused instead on buying up smaller biotech companies that have developed promising drug compounds.

Under this "buy not build" model, biotech companies that have drugs in their pipelines to treat cancer, muscular dystrophy, and other diseases are ripe for buyouts by the larger companies that are not as successful in their discoveries.[26] The consulting firm Bain recently conducted a study that showed that the top pharmaceutical corporations were earning more than 70 percent of their sales from medicines that were developed by someone else, usually smaller companies more narrowly focused on a limited number of research projects.[27] As Bernard Munos, a pharmaceutical industry consultant, told the journal *Nature* in 2016, "Most (pharmaceutical corporations) do not produce enough innovation to grow. In fact, half of them are shrinking. They try to mitigate this by escalating prices, which is dangerous. I think industry is misjudging the anger that its practices are creating."[28] Also in 2016, one pharma CEO, Dr. Leonard Schleifer of Regeneron Pharmaceuticals, conceded the point: "The real reason we're not liked, in my opinion, is because, we as an industry, have used price hikes to cover up the gaps in innovation."[29]

An example of this dynamic is the massively profitable hepatitis C medicines (discussed in chapters 1 and 2), which have been priced out of the range of patients such as Sarah Jackson. The drugs were developed by the biotech firm Pharmasset. (As I explore further in chapter 14, these hepatitis C medicines are among the majority of important medicines whose late-stage development was built on a foundation of basic research that was largely government-funded.) In 2011, the larger corporation Gilead bought up Pharmasset and the patent rights to its wonder drugs for $11 billion.[30] It was a big price tag, but the high prices of Sovaldi and Harvoni are allowing Gilead to make up that investment very quickly. Even while the pharmaceutical industry aggressively promotes itself as an innovator, occasionally a corporate executive will reveal the true nature of the current business model. "We're not going to put our money in-house if there's a better investment vehicle outside," the chief operating officer (COO) of GlaxoSmithKline told the *Wall Street Journal*.[31]

THE CURRENT SYSTEM WASTES BILLIONS ON DRUG MARKETING

As we have seen, the justification claimed by the pharmaceutical industry for patent monopoly protections and the resulting high prices for drugs centers on its need to fund research and development of new medicines. Conspicuously absent from that justification is any mention of the money the industry spends to sell and market its drugs. But those costs are not absent from the corporate balance sheets. In fact, the sales and marketing expenses of the pharmaceutical corporations are significantly larger than their investments in research.

The exact figures vary from corporation to corporation and from year to year and are often not fully revealed in public, but the overall picture is of an industry that spends nearly twice as much on selling its existing products than it does on researching new ones.[1] Here is one example: in 2013, Johnson & Johnson spent $8.2 billion on research and development, and $17.5 billion on sales and marketing.[2] Another example: in 2014, Pfizer spent $8.4 billion on research and development, and $14.1 billion on sales and marketing. That same year, the Pfizer research and development costs were also exceeded by the money it spent paying dividends to its stockholders and the financial maneuver of buying back its own shares of stock.[3]

The United States is one of just three countries in the world that allows direct-to-consumer advertising of drugs—New Zealand and Brazil are the others.[4] Pharmaceutical corporations spend over $5 billion per year for such ads, and they do so for one reason: they work.[5] Commercials for branded drugs have been proven to motivate patients to ask their doctors about the drugs being promoted and often to directly request a prescription for them.[6] In addition, patients who see drug advertising are more likely to ask their physician for the more expensive branded versions, even when there are generic alternatives.[7] And doctors are more likely to prescribe the branded drugs when their patients ask about them.[8]

In the United States, the Medicare system spent $4 billion in 2013 on branded and heavily marketed medicines for heartburn and high cholesterol, even though far cheaper alternatives were available.[9] In 2015, physician members of the American Medical Association voted to support a U.S. ban on direct-to-consumer advertising, saying "a growing proliferation of ads is driving demand for expensive treatments despite the clinical effectiveness of less costly alternatives."[10]

Many of us in the United States are weary of the seemingly endless drug commercials on U.S. television, online, or in glossy advertisements in magazines and newspapers—1.3 million of these TV ads are broadcast annually with well over 100 airing each and every hour, which together cost the industry more than $4 billion.[11] So it may come as a shock to learn that these commercials do not represent the biggest marketing investments of the drug companies. Those companies actually spend six times more on pitching their products to those who write the prescriptions than they do on advertising directly to consumers.[12] The marketing-to-prescribers approaches include a practice the industry calls "detailing"—face-to-face meetings with health care providers, which are accompanied by gifts and meals, free samples, and sponsorship of professional meetings and journals.

A 2007 report in the *New England Journal of Medicine* showed the remarkable penetration of these efforts in the United States: 83 percent of physicians reported receiving food and beverages in the workplace from drug companies; 78 percent reported being given drug samples by a manufacturer representative; over one-third reported receiving reimbursements for the costs associated with professional meetings or continuing medical education; and more than one-quarter reported receiving payments for consulting, speaking, or enrolling patients in trials.[13] Some of the most egregious excesses of the marketing process have recently been curbed by the industry and physicians, but the overall intensity of the sales job remains at a high level. Drug corporations now deploy a whopping 72,000 pharmaceutical sales representatives in the United States alone.[14]

Similar to direct-to-consumer advertising, the marketing to physicians has proven to be an effective strategy for pharmaceutical corporations. A recent study analyzing data from 12 drug companies, more than 330,000 physicians, and nearly 1 billion prescriptions found that physicians who received drug company payments were significantly more likely to prescribe the drug sold by that company.[15] Another study showed the physicians who accepted free meals from drug companies were far more likely to prescribe brand-name drugs than the generic versions.[16] Giving out free drug samples have been shown to increase the likelihood that, after the freebies run out, physicians will prescribe the medicine even if it is inappropriate or more expensive than alternatives.[17] Add it all up, and that marketing contributes mightily to Americans' spending an extra $24 billion each year as a result of bypassing cheaper generics for higher-price brand-name drugs.[18]

THE CURRENT SYSTEM COMPROMISES PHYSICIAN INTEGRITY AND LEADS TO UNETHICAL CORPORATE BEHAVIOR

In chapter 7, I discussed how the pharmaceutical industry spends billions of dollars each year marketing its products to health care providers, particularly physicians.[1] Beyond the tens of thousands of company salespersons deployed to directly market their products to physicians, pharmaceutical and medical device companies also pay a full two-thirds of the costs of continuing medical education in medical schools and teaching hospitals. Predictably, the content of the programming often reflects that influence.[2] Drug company marketing also reaches into the level of direct care. One example of such controversial industry expenditures is paying providers to participate in "patient adherence programs," which aim to encourage patients to take branded medicines.[3]

There is no mystery to why pharmaceutical companies want to cultivate physicians and other care providers: these individuals write the prescriptions that dictate the company's bottom line. As a Federal Trade Commission report said, in the current medical system, "the consumer who pays does not choose, and the physician who chooses does not pay."[4]

But there is another motivation as well. Surveys show that patients do not trust drug companies (in 2015, 74 percent believed pharmaceutical companies put profits before people) but that they do trust doctors (78 percent of Americans reported feeling positively about physicians).[5] By winning over physicians to their products, pharmaceutical companies are purchasing some of that caregiver goodwill.

To many in the health care community, this is an alarming situation. The physician Ben Goldacre, in his book *Bad Pharma: How Drug Companies Mislead Doctors and Harm Patients*, explains to non-physicians why the drug industry's central role in funding and shaping continuing medical education is so impactful:

> Doctors spend forty years practicing medicine, with very little formal education after their initial training. Medicine changes completely in four decades, and as they try to keep up, doctors are bombarded with information: from ads that misrepresent the benefits and risks of new medicines; from sales reps who spy on patients' confidential prescribing records; from colleagues who are quietly paid by drug companies; from "teaching" that is sponsored by the industry; from independent "academic" journal articles that are quietly written by drug company employees; and worse.[6]

Citing the psychological research that has firmly established that even small gifts influence decision making, some leading voices in the medical field have called for the money to stop flowing from the drug corporations to physicians.[7] A 2008 editorial in the *Journal of the American Medical Association* made the reasoning plain: "The profession of medicine, in every aspect—clinical, education, and research—has been inundated with profound influence from the pharmaceutical and medical device industries. This has occurred because physicians have allowed it to happen, and it is time to stop."[8] Similar concern among the public caused the U.S. Congress to pass in 2010 the Physician Payment Sunshine Act, which requires that drug and medical device companies report their financial relationships with physicians.[9]

Beyond the influence of the pharmaceutical industry on the clinical practice of medicine, the corporate influence on medical research has caused just as much concern. A 2006 survey of department chairs in accredited medical schools and teaching hospitals revealed that almost two-thirds of the chairs had financial relationships with the pharmaceutical and medical device industry. Industry roles for the department chairs included their serving as consultants, members of corporate scientific advisory boards, and paid speakers.[10] According to Daniel Wikkler, Harvard ethics and health professor, these esteemed academic physicians are acting as "surrogate sales staff," and entire academic departments have reputations of being "owned" by particular pharmaceutical companies.[11]

A 2007 survey found that over half of academic life science researchers had a relationship with the pharmaceutical industry.[12] That relationship sometimes comes with strings attached: many researchers who received pharmaceutical industry gifts reported that the corporation requested a prepublication review of articles or reports stemming from the use of the gift and sought promises that biomaterials provided would not be used for research that would compete with company products.[13] As for the influential journals themselves, a former editor of the prestigious British medical journal the *Lancet* has said, "Journals have devolved into information-laundering operations for the pharmaceutical industry."[14] Editors of several other prominent journals have agreed with him.[15]

As with their marketing to clinical physicians, the motivation of the pharmaceutical industry for these marketing investments in the research field is clear: they help the corporate bottom line. Reviews of corporate-sponsored medical studies compared to non-sponsored studies show that the corporate-sponsored versions were significantly more likely to report that the drug studied was effective and beneficial, and less likely to find negative effects caused by the drug.[16] On the level of the individual researchers, industry-sponsored physicians and scientists have been shown to report disproportionately industry-favorable results.[17] As one former pharmaceutical industry executive plainly stated, this is exactly the desired outcome: "It is to industry's advantage to selectively support particular researchers whose point of view supports marketing goals, and to encourage selective publication of articles."[18]

The design of industry-sponsored studies often benefits those marketing goals, too. Clinical trials are disproportionately industry-sponsored, and those trials routinely compare the company drug to only a placebo rather than to a similar medicine. That means the results of the study do not reveal whether the new medicine is actually better than existing products already available. The resulting "better than nothing" standard sets a very low bar for the studied drug and does not yield the information that would be most valuable to physicians, who need to decide which medicine to prescribe.[19]

There are other significant problems with industry-sponsored clinical trials. To Ben Goldacre, the most concerning is the widespread failure to share the results of trials that are not positive for the company. "For me, missing data is the key to this whole story," Goldacre says. "It poisons the well for everybody. If proper trials are never done, if trials with negative results are withheld, then we can simply not know the true effects of the treatments we use. . . . With missing data, we are all in this together, and we are all misled."[20] In addition, some clinical trials sponsored by drug companies occur after the drug has already been approved. These trials are known as Phase IV trials. Although there can be legitimate research reasons to conduct these trials, the goals of these post-approval studies often appear less focused on actual research than on promoting the product through paying clinical doctors to use it on patients.[21]

One particularly disturbing example of the impact of industry-sponsored research was the delayed reporting of the dangers of erythropoetin-stimulating agents (ESAs), used to treat anemia in cancer patients. Early industry-sponsored research in the 1990s showed ESAs had benefits, but later reports by independent researchers showed the drugs actually significantly increased the risk of patient death. While none of the industry-sponsored research reported these major problems, 90 percent of studies not funded by pharmaceutical corporations did.[22]

Undoubtedly, some of the purchased industry influence on reported research results is working at the subconscious level. But some of the impact is not subtle at all. Two high-profile articles published together in the *Journal of the American Medical Association* in 2008 outlined how Merck may have intentionally misrepresented the risks of its medicines in articles reporting research on its products. Those articles were apparently written by Merck employees but published under the names of academic researchers who had had little to do with the studies.[23] Corporate-hired ghostwriters regularly author research articles that promote drugs manufactured by the company, yet the articles appear under the names of academic physicians. The ghostwriting tactic has also been used by Eli Lilly and GlaxoSmithKline, among others.[24]

The deep and wide influence of the pharmaceutical industry on health care is no secret. Multiple books have been published decrying the situation, several written by esteemed authors who are faculty at Harvard Medical School or were once editors in chief of the *New England Journal of Medicine*.[25] One of these authors is Marcia Angell, who was the editor of the *New England Journal of Medicine* in 2000 when the journal published an article studying an antidepressant. The author of the article, who was the chair of a university psychiatry department, had reportedly made over $500,000 in a single year consulting for corporations that manufactured antidepressants. A concerned Dr. Angell decided to write an editorial to accompany the article. The editorial was entitled, "Is Academic Medicine for Sale?"[26] After the editorial was published, a physician from Detroit responded with a three-sentence letter to the editor. "Is academic medicine for sale?" repeated Thomas J. Ruane, MD. "No. The current owner is quite happy with it."[27]

Of course, it is not unusual for multinational corporations to engage in aggressive lobbying and marketing. But, as U.S. Senator Debbie Stabenow (D-MI) has said, "'Medicine is different. It's not like buying a car or tennis shoes or peanut butter."[28] The World Health Organization has called this tension "an inherent conflict of interest between the legitimate business goals of (medicine) manufacturers and social, medical, and economic needs."[29] As we see in chapter 16, there is a long history of societies treating medicines as public goods, protected from the scarcity and profiteering that can affect access to less essential consumer goods.

In contrast, for the pharmaceutical industry the pursuit of profits has often transcended any reasonable definition of the "legitimate business goals" the WHO refers to. As the watchdog organization Transparency International wrote in 2016, "Within the health sector, pharmaceuticals stands out as sub-sector that is particularly prone to corruption. There are abundant examples globally that display how corruption in the pharmaceutical sector endangers positive health outcomes."[30]

Many examples of this were chronicled in a 2010 study by the U.S. nonprofit Public Citizen, which found that the pharmaceutical industry is far and away the largest defrauder of U.S. federal and state governments.[31] Pharmaceutical corporations have been cited for dozens of major violations of the U.S. False Claims Act, the Anti-Kickback Statute, the Foreign Corrupt Practices Act, and multiple state laws prohibiting Medicaid fraud.[32] In the twenty-year period ending in 2010, pharmaceutical companies entered into 165 civil or criminal settlements with federal and state governments, and the number of citations showed steady annual increases at both the federal and state levels.[33] The total settlements in that period added up to $19.81 billion.[34]

The four biggest offenders over this period—GlaxoSmithKline, Pfizer, Eli Lilly, and Schering-Plough—were all fined more than $1 billion each.[35] In 2012, Pfizer settled charges that it had bribed health officials in multiple countries, and GlaxoSmithKline was fined for failing to report the adverse effects of one of its medicines.[36] Several companies were cited for overcharging state Medicaid programs, sometimes collecting as much as twelve times the legal cost of their medicines.[37] Some were punished for paying off potential generic competitors.[38]

In addition, Purdue Pharma was criminally sanctioned for its role in falsely underplaying the addiction risks of its painkiller drug Oxycontin, and its aggressive and ethically suspect marketing of the drug has been cited as a chief trigger of an ongoing opioid and heroin epidemic in the United States.[39] (Not coincidentally, the pharmaceutical industry was at the same time leading the opposition to the legalization of medical marijuana, as studies have shown that medical marijuana legalization leads to decreased prescribing of painkillers, anxiety medication, and other staples of corporate pharmaceutical product lines.[40]) An ongoing case against Novartis, in which the company is accused of funneling kickbacks to prescribers through thousands of supposed "educational" meetings where doctors were wined and dined, may lead to a multibillion dollar fine.[41] In 2016, pharma sales representatives were arrested and charged in New York with violating federal antikickback laws. The allegation is that the representatives from Insys used sham educational meetings as a cover for paying physicians to prescribe highly addictive opioids.[42] Also in 2016, the South African drug maker Aspen Pharmacare was fined by Italian authorities for blocking supplies of several cancer drugs, a tactic the company employed to negotiate huge price increases.[43]

For drug companies, the most commonly cited ethical offense involves a tactic called "off-label promotion." Physicians are allowed to prescribe drugs off label, meaning prescribing them for a different disease or type of patient than has been approved by regulatory agencies. But in the United States and other countries, pharmaceutical corporations are strictly prohibited from promoting these off-label uses of their products because those uses have not been analyzed for possibly dangerous effects.[44] Nevertheless, they do just that. For example, Pfizer was charged in 2009 with illegally promoting off-label uses of the pain medicine Bextra, which was later pulled from the market for safety reasons.[45]

Some of the many recent big-dollar fines levied for off-label promotions include the record-setting $12 billion settlement by GlaxoSmithKline regarding allegations it illegally promoted its antidepressant Paxil for use in adolescents, the $2.3 billion settlement by Pfizer regarding claims it illegally promoted drugs off-label, and the $1.4 billion payment by Eli Lilly after claims it illegally promoted its antipsychotic drug Zyprexa—even to the point of training its sales persons in how to avoid legal requirements.[46] "Marketing departments of many drug companies don't respect any boundaries of professionalism or the law," according to Jerry Avorn, a professor at Harvard Medical School. "The Pfizer and Lilly cases (for example) involved the illegal promotion of drugs that have been shown to cause substantial harm and death to patients."[47] One study analyzed the impact of corporate mismarketing alleged in five prominent cases (involving the drugs Vioxx, Avandia, Bextra, OxyContin, and Zyprexa), and estimated the annual costs to society caused by the resulting sickness and death. The resulting figure of $27 billion a year in cost is an amount roughly equal to the industry's claimed research investments over the same period.[48]

Government officials admit to frustration that the many fines do not deter off-label promotion. One physician complains that the punishments "are nothing more than parking tickets."[49] Even multibillion dollar penalties do not measure up to much more than a fraction of the annual profits of these companies.[50] And much of that profit is being earned through the very practices that are being prosecuted; studies suggest that one out of every five prescriptions is written for off-label use.[51]

Beyond off-label promotion, the pharmaceutical industry has aggressively engaged in a practice known as "disease mongering," sometimes called the more polite term "condition branding."[52] The approach is to take unpleasant but common aspects of the human condition and label them as medical diseases that corporate drug products can address. Examples of this technique are numerous: shyness was rebranded as "social anxiety disorder" to market the antidepressant Paxil, premenstrual syndrome became the ominous-sounding "premenstrual dysphoric disorder," which Prozac was promoted to address, and heartburn was upgraded to gastro-esophageal reflux disease, which Zantac stood ready to remedy.[53] The industry has come under heavy criticism for its role in what many believe to be a significant overdiagnosis of attention deficit–hyperactivity disorder in children and adults in the United States[54]

The iconic example of disease mongering is the transformation by the pharmaceutical industry of impotence into "erectile dysfunction," accomplished by saturation ad campaigns and testimonies from paid researchers and physicians. The drugs promoted to treat what the industry labeled "E.D." have become blockbuster sellers.[55] That success soon inspired an effort to create a parallel "hypoaffective sexual desire disorder" for women. Despite the lack of any scientifically established norm for sexual desire or any evidence that low libido is an actual medical condition, pharmaceutical corporations pushed for approval to market testosterone patches and gels to address the situation.[56]

Beginning in the mid-2000s, hypoaffective sexual desire disorder was exhaustively promoted in industry-funded continuing medical education (CME) courses. Those courses drove home some commercially favorable messages: the disorder was common and underdiagnosed, women may not even be aware they have the condition, and clinicians should initiate conversations on the topic with their female patients.[57] One CME module even said that women who were highly interested in sex, just not with their current partner, may still be appropriately diagnosed as having a "situational" form of the disorder.[58] Not surprisingly, a *Journal of Medical Ethics* review of the campaign around hypoaffective sexual desire disorder called it "inventing a disease" and "a typical example of the medicalization of a normal state."[59]

The pharmaceutical industry has also been accused of unethical behavior for its use of what seems at first glance to be a positive practice: medicine donation programs, sometimes known as patient-assistance programs. "The glorified term, 'patient assistance program' is nothing but a marketing strategy," an Indian medical ethicists told the *New York Times*.[60] There are multiple examples to back up that statement. Novartis has been sharply criticized for giving away far less of its cancer drug Gleevec than it had promised and for then threatening to stop donations in countries where generic versions were permitted.[61] Novartis also pushed the recipients of its donations to lobby their governments to buy the drug at high prices and to oppose generic competition, a common request made to individual patients and patient groups who receive drug company donations.[62] Many desperate patients and families are willing to comply with company requests, but are disappointed to learn that these programs are much less extensive than industry rhetoric suggests, especially since Medicare, Medicaid, and veterans' program enrollees are not eligible and many programs require private insurance coverage.[63]

Insurers and industry observers say the leveraging of drug donations for brand promotion and to discourage generics has the effect of driving up the cost of medicines—and the profits of the companies.[64] In 2016, *Bloomberg News* conducted an investigation into such programs, concluding that they are a public relations–focused "billion-dollar system in which charitable giving is, in effect, a very profitable form of investing for drug companies."[65] Later that year, a whistleblower lawsuit filed by a former Celgene employee claimed that the company was using its donations to patient charities as a mechanism to ensure that Medicare covered its drugs, thus directing billions of dollars in payments to the company.[66]

This dispiritingly long list of ethical problems in the pharmaceutical industry cannot conclude without a mention of the financial machinations that huge pharma corporations use to avoid paying taxes, particularly in the United States. In 2015, the U.S. pharmaceutical giant Pfizer announced it would pursue the largest ever "tax inversion," a strategy in which a corporation merges with a foreign competitor to relocate its legally defined headquarters to a country with lower taxes. In 2014, U.S. President Barack Obama called inversion companies "corporate deserters."[67] The Pfizer plan to merge with Dublin-based Allergan and shift its headquarters to low-tax Ireland drew sharp criticisms. "The Pfizer-Allergan deal will be the biggest inversion yet, and it is nothing short of a disgrace," wrote John Cassidy in the *New Yorker* in late 2015. "Drug companies like Pfizer have long benefitted from taxpayer-funded research carried out under the auspices of organizations like the NIH and the National Science Foundation. Now, Pfizer is seeking to avoid paying the taxes that are due on its profits."[68]

The Pfizer-Allergan merger was eventually abandoned. But the philosophy it represented is alive and well. Even as U.S.-based pharmaceutical corporations rely on taxpayer-supported research and high-price high-volume government drug purchases (see chapters 16 and 17), they still relentlessly pursue methods to avoid paying U.S. taxes. Pfizer has stashed $74 billion in profits overseas to avoid U.S. taxes, and Merck has $60 billion similarly tucked away.[69] Gilead, the U.S. company whose blockbuster hepatitis C medicine was created using U.S.-funded research and is purchased primarily by U.S. government agencies, has transferred the patent for the medicine to an Irish subsidiary.[70] As Frank Clemente, executive director of Americans for Tax Fairness, said, ""Gilead is making a fortune selling essential drugs to the very government and taxpayers that helped pay to develop them, and then dodging taxes on the resulting profits."[71]

9

MEDICINES ARE PRICED AT WHATEVER THE MARKET WILL BEAR

We have seen that in late summer 2015 medicine prices suddenly became headline news in the United States (see chapter 2). It is worth looking a little more into the background and context of this phenomenon. The drug that triggered the media attention is called Daraprim, the standard treatment for the parasitic infection toxoplasmosis, a condition that is particularly dangerous for patients suffering from AIDS and cancer. Daraprim, which had no competing product on the market, had been recently purchased by a startup company called Turing Pharmaceuticals, run by a thirty-two year-old former hedge fund manager named Martin Shkreli. After purchasing the rights to the drug, Turing and Shkreli immediately raised the price of Daraprim from $13.50 a tablet to $750.[1]

The price hike, the company, and Shkreli himself were fiercely criticized. The criticism came first from physicians and care providers, and then from social media commenters. Ultimately, politicians, including presidential candidates from both major U.S. parties, joined in.[2] Even the PhRMA, in a statement on its Twitter account, distanced itself from the price hike: "@TuringPharma does not represent the values of @PhRMA member companies."[3]

Yet it does. In response to the PhRMA statement, a Turing spokesperson pointed out that its actions were far from unprecedented in the pharmaceutical industry.[4] And U.S. Representative Elijah Cummings (D-MD), ranking member of a congressional committee studying drug pricing, said of the Turing approach, "These tactics are not limited to a few bad apples, but are prominent throughout the industry."[5]

The abrupt spike in the price of Daraprim was just an extreme example of the deadly dynamics of the pharmaceutical industry, in which corporate monopolies have exclusive control over products that are necessary for the survival of millions. The result is prices that are set at whatever the market will bear, and it is inevitable that the market will bear enormous prices when lives are on the line.[6] As noted in a November 2015 article that appeared in the *Economist* following the news of the Daraprim pricing, the for-profit nature of the medicine system all but compels corporations to gouge its customers: "The shareholders of a drugmaker expect it to charge as much as it can get away with; and since many drugs, for as long as their patent is in force, have no close competitors, the health systems and insurers they sell to may have little choice but to pay whatever they are asked for."[7]

In other words, the 5,000 percent overnight price increase of Daraprim caused a whiplash for the media and politicians, but more public relations–savvy pharmaceutical corporations routinely help themselves to less dramatic but still sizable price increases. In the United States in 2015, the same year that Daraprim earned headlines, prices for branded medicines quietly rose almost 15 percent on average, more than seven times the rate of inflation.[8] Sixty of those drugs doubled in price or more, and twenty of them quadrupled in price.[9] This type of annual increase is the norm; analysts from Morgan Stanley have reported that drug prices have been rising at overall rates of 12 percent annually for years.[10] In 2016, the director of the U.S. Centers for Medicaid and Medicare Services said that he had once defended the pharmaceutical industry against being defined by a few bad actors but that he eventually was forced to admit that large price increases were both pervasive and unsustainable.[11]

The story behind these steady increases, and the original prices set by the corporate medicine patent-holders, reveals why the prices of medicines are so high. Medicine prices are determined by a highly unusual process that has no relation to the normal considerations of manufacturers or retailers in competitive markets. As the U.S. Department of Health and Human Services bluntly stated in a 2016 report, "In reality, the prices charged for drugs are unrelated to their development costs. Drug manufacturers set prices to maximize profits."[12] The medicine pricing system also does not bear any resemblance to markets in which the consumer has the option to decline to purchase the product. In truth, Assistant Secretary-General Marie-Paule Kieny of the World Health Organization has admitted, "Amid public outcry, political battles and media articles, no one seems to understand how, exactly, medicines prices are set."[13]

But there are some clues. Analyses of the corporate medicine price-setting process have shown that, when a company arrives at the price to be charged, neither research and development investments nor the cost of manufacturing medicines is considered. Instead, corporate executives conduct detailed research into the maximum amount they can charge without causing insurers and governments to refuse to pay for the medicine and physicians to shy away from prescribing it.[14] Sometimes, when demand spikes, those calculations are quickly adjusted. For example, a recent surge in opioid addictions in the United States has been quickly followed by as much as a seventeenfold increase in the price of a drug that can reverse an opioid overdose.[15]

The *Wall Street Journal* report on the Pfizer cancer drug pricing process (see chapter 4), made no bones about the overarching goal of the corporate deliberation: Pfizer wanted to be very certain that it was not leaving any money on the table.[16] That is why medicines for deadly diseases are sometimes priced at six hundred times the cost to make them.[17] And that is why, in the United States, where the government Medicare program is barred from negotiating the price of the drugs it pays for, medicines are priced more than double what is charged in similar countries that do negotiate.[18]

One illustration of this what-the-market-will-bear pricing dynamic is the cost of the patent-protected hepatitis C drugs Sovaldi and Harvoni, which we have learned (see chapter 1) have been priced out of the reach of U.S. Medicaid patients such as Sarah Jackson. The corporate pharmaceutical pricing process is typically hidden from public view, but the U.S. Senate Finance Committee conducted an eighteen-month investigation into how Gilead Sciences arrived at the hepatitis C medicine prices. The Senate committee reviewed evidence compiled from 20,000 pages of company documents, Medicaid records, and dozens of interviews with experts.[19] The investigation found that, in arriving at the $84,000 price tag for a twelve-week course of Sovaldi, the corporation did not consider at all the manufacturing cost of about $100 for that course of the medicine.[20] Nor did Gilead concern itself with the need of patients such as Sarah Jackson to access the medicine. In fact, the Senate investigation found that the company executives were "fully aware" that the target price would put the medicine out of reach for many.[21]

Instead, Gilead looked at the $36,000 treatment price identified as a target by the Sovaldi developer Pharmasset, which Gilead had purchased in 2012, and decided it could do better.[22] Almost $50,000 better, as it turned out. The company considered the remarkable effectiveness of the medicine whose rights it had purchased, looked closely at what it felt the market would bear, and set a price that was 617 times greater than its manufacturing costs. Senator Ron Wyden (D-OR) of the Senate Finance Committee summed up the corporate process uncovered by the investigation:

> Gilead pursued a calculated scheme for pricing and marketing its Hepatitis C drug based on one primary goal, maximizing revenue, regardless of the human consequences. There was no concrete evidence in emails, meeting minutes or presentations that basic financial matters such as R&D costs or the multi-billion dollar acquisition of Pharmasset, the drug's first developer, factored into how Gilead set the price. Gilead knew these prices would put treatment out of the reach of millions and cause extraordinary problems for Medicare and Medicaid, but still the company went ahead.[23]

That is sharp criticism from a high-level official. But Gilead saw all this coming, and the company executives bolstered themselves for the inevitable condemnation of the price of the medicine. After the drug was released, one company vice president offered a pep talk in an internal e-mail. 'Let's hold our position whatever competitors do, or whatever the headlines," he wrote in late 2013. "Let's not fold to advocacy pressure in 2014."[24] That advice was heeded, and Gilead has reaped the rewards for it. In twenty-one months after the medicine was introduced, the company collected $20.6 billion in revenue for it.[25]

Another disturbing medicine price-setting example, this one with even more widespread deadly impact, is the cost of lifesaving vaccines. As we have seen in chapter 3, the young boy Ahmed and millions more like him die each year from diseases that could have been prevented by vaccinations. One of the world's leading providers of childhood vaccines, Médecins Sans Frontières/Doctors Without Borders, issued a 2015 report entitled "The Right Shot: Bringing Down Barriers to Affordable and Adapted Vaccines," chronicling the dizzying 7,000 percent increase in vaccine package pricing from 2011 to 2014.[26]

The vaccine price hikes were caused by several factors. First, a limited number of vaccine manufacturers means that large companies such as GlaxoSmithKline, Pfizer, and Merck can corner the market with duopolies and oligopolies, keeping prices high until a low-cost competitor can enter the market.[27] Second, the industry fiercely guards the secrecy of the actual prices it charges to the health systems of individual countries, even forcing purchasers to sign price confidentiality agreements. When MSF asked for pricing information for its report, the multinational corporate vaccine manufacturers refused.[28] That corporate strategy quite intentionally puts individual countries at a disadvantage when negotiating vaccine prices. What little is known about vaccine pricing reveals the benefits of that leverage: corporations are charging some countries prices that are at least twelve to sixteen times the manufacturing cost.[29]

The result is more medicine pricing at the limit of what a market will bear—"as high as the purchaser will tolerate," in the words of the MSF report—even if that means radically different prices from one country to the next.[30] And even if that means that children such as Ahmed die. "Many children living in middle-income countries are not benefitting from new, lifesaving vaccines, as a result of irrational and unaffordable pricing policies," the MSF report concludes.[31] As noted in chapter 3, in 2016, the two producers of the pneumococcal vaccine announced they would lower the prices they charged humanitarian organizations, reducing but not eliminating the gaps in vaccine availability.[32]

Vaccines and hepatitis C medicines are certainly not the only examples of pricing that exploits patients' desperate need to obtain medicine that will stave off misery or death. Just a partial review of the market in 2015 demonstrates that. For example, Valeant Pharmaceuticals doubled the price of over a dozen drugs that year, including a 720 percent increase for a key heart medicine.[33] In response to criticism by hospitals and lawmakers, Valeant promised to provide discounts, but those discounts represented only a fraction of the price hikes.[34] In 2014, Valeant raised the price of a lead poisoning drug by 2,700 percent over the course of the single year.[35] Pfizer raised its prices for 133 drugs in 2015, most by 10 percent or more and some by as much as 84 percent.[36]

Also in 2015, Pfizer and its partner Flynn Pharma were accused by a UK regulatory agency of abusing their dominant role in the epilepsy drug market by charging an "excessive and unfair" price on an anti-epilepsy drug.[37] Some of the Pfizer price hikes, including on big sellers such as the pain medicine Lyrica and the erectile dysfunction drug Viagra, reflect a common pattern in drug pricing: these medicines are set to go off patent soon, so the company is squeezing its fading monopoly for every dollar while it can.[38]

Also in 2015, GlaxoSmithKline and Merck hiked their drug prices as well, and people with diabetes endured a 36 percent price increase from Eli Lilly for Humalog, a fast-acting insulin.[39] The price for a kidney disease medicine jumped 2,000 percent, and the prices of two blood pressure drugs went up 600 percent.[40] Exciting news in 2013 of the development of two new badly needed TB drugs was dampened by the prices set by their manufacturers, Johnson & Johnson and Otsuka. The corporations have set the prices at levels that are dozens of times the manufacturing costs. As a result, the TB medicines are out of reach for those who need them the most; only one in every fifty patients who need the medicine is getting it.[41]

This what-the-market-will-bear dynamic is well demonstrated by the response of corporate patent-holders when they conclude that the market may not actually tolerate the prices they set. For example, when the U.S. government threatened in 2001 to allow the generic manufacturing of the Bayer patented drug ciprofloxacin (see chapter 18), the company quickly cut the price of the medicine in half.[42] In 2004, Abbot made an even larger price reduction when pressured by the U.S. government on the cost of an AIDS medicine.[43] When prominent oncologists wrote a 2012 *New York Times* opinion column saying they would not prescribe the drug Zaltrap because of its price, the drug's manufacturer Sanofi quickly lowered its price by 50 percent.[44]

But those price reductions are the exception. When medicines are essential to health, patients and government health programs have reliably shown themselves to be willing to pay prices with enormous markups. As U.S. Senator Charles Grassley (R-IA) said at the conclusion of the lengthy investigation into the monopoly pricing of Sovaldi by Gilead at $1,000 per pill, "This might be an example that received the most attention in some time, but it won't be the last."[45]

PHARMACEUTICAL CORPORATIONS REAP HISTORY-MAKING PROFITS

If you are a pharmaceutical company CEO, congratulations! You have won the corporate equivalent of the lottery. Consider your bulletproof business plan. Governments conduct the riskiest and most time-consuming research and development in your industry, and then you are awarded monopolies on the products of that research. Your customers' lives may depend on obtaining your product, so they are often forced to pay whatever price you decide to charge. Even better, governments are reliable bulk purchasers of your product, and some government programs are even prohibited by law from negotiating down your asking price.

Given this sweet arrangement, it is no wonder that the pharmaceutical industry is one of the most profitable business sectors in modern history. In 2013, five major pharmaceutical companies made a profit margin of 20 percent or more, and several regularly have profit margins of greater than 30 percent.[1] Every business aims to make a profit, but let us consider those numbers in context. Pharmaceutical corporations make a return on their assets that is more than double the average of all the Fortune 500 companies.[2] In the past decade, the top ten pharmaceutical companies made more in profits than the rest of the Fortune 500 companies combined.[3] Year after year, rankings of the most profitable industries reliably put pharmaceutical corporations at the very top or close to the top, higher than legendary money makers such as banks and oil companies.[4]

I discuss later (chapters 16, 17, and 22) how longtime moral and legal traditions suggest that medicines research, manufacturing, and distribution should not be dependent on a for-profit scheme. But even many who believe a profit motive has a place in our medicines system are convinced that the level of profits in the pharmaceutical industry rises far above what is reasonable and appropriate, especially given the human cost incurred.[5]

Pfizer, the world's largest pharmaceutical company, provides a good example of the cash-flush nature of the industry. In 2013, Pfizer reported a 42 percent profit margin, a return that the BBC characterized as "eye-watering," part of a two-year stretch during which the company generated over $9 billion annually in net profits.[6] Do you remember (chapter 3) that Ahmed and millions of children die each year because of a lack of affordable vaccines? One of the top Pfizer product lines is vaccines, and the corporation earns more than $17 million each day in sales from its pneumonia vaccine alone.[7]

Pfizer is a prominent member of PhRMA, which spends significant industry money putting forth the argument that its member companies take enormous business risks. "Biopharmaceutical R&D is an extremely complex process and failure is more common than success," according to PhRMA.[8] But that argument is undermined by the year-after-year industry record of world-leading profits. As Alan Sager, Boston University health economist, puts it, "If you went to Las Vegas with $1,000 and routinely came back with $1400, could your family accuse you of gambling?"[9]

What do pharmaceutical corporations do with their billions in windfall profits? Although industry public relations would have us believe the companies put that money into research and development, many highly profitable corporations have reduced their research investments in recent years. Marianna Mazzucato, an economist, says this is a predictable result of a system that allows private industry to benefit from government investments in research— called free-riding.[10] So, instead of ramping up their research and development, pharmaceutical corporations spend billions in financial maneuvers such as buying back shares of their own stock.[11] Pfizer again provides a good example of this practice. Between 2003 and

2012, the company spent $59 billion of its profits in stock buybacks.[12] In 2014 alone, Pfizer spent almost $12 billion to buy back its own shares and to pay dividends to its shareholders—financial transactions that added up to almost 50 percent more than the company spent on research and development.[13]

Why do Pfizer and other drug companies buy back their own stock? To the public, corporate CEOs provide one answer. When he announced a $10 billion stock buyback in 2011, Ian Read, the Pfizer CEO, said the plan was "a testament to our continued commitment to enhancing shareholder value and to our continued confidence in the business."[14] In other words, pharmaceutical stock is so valuable, we want more of it for ourselves.

But in truth, stock buybacks are conducted because they benefit the two most powerful forces in pharmaceutical industry: shareholders and top executives. First, stock buybacks lift the company stock price (note the reference to "enhancing shareholder value" by Read), which makes shareholders happy. Second, buybacks that lift stock values make pharmaceutical company CEOs even happier because their salaries are typically tied to the price of the company stock.[15]

CEOs and other top executives are the big winners in the stock-buyback scheme, which is a core reason why the pay of high-level corporate executives has more than doubled since the early 1990s.[16] Over the course of the 2003–2012 decade, the largest eleven pharmaceutical companies paid their CEOs a combined salary of $1.57 billion.[17] In 2015, the average compensation for CEOs of the large pharma corporations was over $18 million, 71 percent more than the average of other large corporations.[18]

Big profits and big salaries may seem relatively harmless until we consider that millions die because they cannot afford the products these corporations produce. A 2016 analysis published in the *BMJ* (formerly the *British Medical Journal*) tied high drug prices, along with reduced research investments, to the current pharma business model of buying products developed elsewhere and then devoting revenue to rewarding stockholders and top executives.[19] In a 2014 article for the *Harvard Business Review*, the health economist William Lazonick reviewed the status of profits, stock buybacks, and executive pay. He concluded that the data make a mockery of the pharmaceutical industry claim that it needs high profits to fund research and development. "The reality is," Lazonick wrote, "Americans pay high drug prices so that major pharmaceutical companies can boost their stock price and pad executive pay."[20]

Part III

PATENTLY POISONOUS

11

THE FOR-PROFIT MEDICINE ARGUMENTS
ARE PATENTLY FALSE

In 2009, Richard DeGeorge, a University of Kansas business ethics professor, wrote an essay entitled "Two Cheers for the Pharmaceutical Industry."[1] DeGeorge pointed to the contributions of the industry to the development of antibiotics, antihypertensive drugs, and beta-blockers.[2] DeGeorge gave drug discoveries some of the credit for the increase in U.S. life expectancy during the second half of the twentieth century and for the reduced cost from missed workdays due to illness.[3] Although conceding that the industry is "far from perfect"—after all, he did call for just two cheers, not three—DeGeorge delivers an overall positive review: "The pharmaceutical industry as a whole has done a great deal to extend longevity, shorten or make hospital stays unnecessary, and meet the expectations of people for new drugs."[4]

DeGeorge made fair points, especially given that he focused on the accomplishments of the industry on behalf of the residents of high-income nations. But the pharmaceutical corporations hardly need him to stand up for them. Their U.S. trade organization, PhRMA, has an annual budget exceeding $200 million, which it directs to the promotion of the image and interests of its fifty-seven member companies.[5] The U.S. lobbying expenses of the industry for 2015 were $238 million.[6] There is a small army of 1,369 lobbyists working for the industry in Washington, DC, alone.[7] And the U.S. political campaign contributions of the industry have been as high as $50.7 million in a year.[8]

Those investments are enormous, ranking among the highest of any industry in the world.[9] PhRMA government lobbying, and the public relations outreach that accompanies it, projects an image of an industry made up of companies that are in the business of healing. The corporation Johnson & Johnson, for example, promotes a corporate credo that places as its top responsibilities patients and health care providers, its employees, and the communities where the company operates. In the credo, only after all these constituencies are described is there a mention of the corporation shareholders.[10] All major pharmaceutical companies vigorously promote their patient-assistance programs, which provide free or reduced-cost medicines.[11]

This public relations goodwill and the political clout behind it are put to the task of defending the patent monopoly system for medicines. (As Charles Keating, a key figure in the U.S. savings-and-loan political scandal of the 1980s and 1990s said when asked if campaign contributions earned him the support from lawmakers, "I want to say in the most forceful way I can: I certainly hope so."[12]) The core of that defense is that patent monopolies are necessary to spur medicine innovation. Without patents, the argument goes, hard-earned discoveries can be immediately copied and sold to others, so no person or organization will have the incentive to devote the resources needed for research and development of new medicines.[13] Here is how PhRMA makes that case:

> Drug research and development leads to the discovery of tomorrow's life-changing and life-saving new medicines. Biopharmaceutical intellectual property (IP) protections, such as patents and data protection, provide the incentives that spur research and development. They help ensure that the innovative biopharmaceutical companies that have invested in life-saving medicines have an opportunity to justify their investments. . . . At the most fundamental level, IP rights give America's biopharmaceutical research companies a chance to fund research into new treatments for our most costly and challenging diseases.[14]

Sometimes the industry and its defenders use the economics term *free riders* to describe organizations or individuals who benefit unfairly from the research conducted by the pharmaceutical corporations.[15] They contend that free riders—in the form of generic producers—need to be blocked or medicine innovation will be stalled.

Parts of this Big Pharma argument are true. Beginning with laboratory research and proceeding to clinical trials, the development of new medicines is indeed an expensive and time-consuming process. As we have seen (chapter 6), however, the industry-promoted estimates of that cost are significantly exaggerated. Nevertheless, there is no question the process costs hundreds of millions of dollars for each drug, and it is also undeniable that society benefits tremendously from the vigorous and creative development of new medicines.

But embedded in the pharmaceutical industry argument for monopoly patent protections are two important ironies. First, the argument concedes the accuracy of one of the core complaints against the drug corporations: the cost of patented medicines sold for prices as high as $1,000 per pill reflects only the existence of a monopoly, not the cost of manufacturing. As we have seen (chapter 9), even many high-priced medicines are produced for just pennies per dose. When corporations set triple-digit markup prices, those numbers are simply a calculation of the maximum amount the industry believes patients will pay and have no relationship to the actual cost of research and production.[16]

The second core irony is that, even though this patent monopoly argument is advanced by corporations that reap history-making profits (as we have seen in chapter 10), the industry rhetoric is actually quite socialist in nature. After all, patents are nothing more than a government-imposed override of the free markets of generic production, allowing the industry to avoid the competitive markets that have proven to dramatically push down the cost of medicines.[17]

Where the pharmaceutical industry argument fails most dramatically is in the assertion that monopoly medicine patents are necessary to spur research and development. The history of medicine discoveries tells a different story. The most impactful medicines, especially vaccines and lifesaving treatments for infectious diseases and chronic diseases, were usually created outside the patent system, and usually supported by government funding.[18]

In fact, it turns out that private pharmaceutical corporations that talk about free enterprise turn to governments to prop up their business model. As we see later (chapter 15), these corporations rely on government funding for pharmaceutical research, which allows them to devote more of their resources to advertising and marketing. And those same corporations count on government dollars coming their way on the back end of their sales process, with government health programs serving as the top purchasers of patented medicines. As one industry commentator put it, the pharmaceutical industry is like the Wizard of Oz—hiding behind a false image as innovators and free market success stories.[19]

So, when it comes to medicines, taxpayers in the United States and other research-supporting countries are the very opposite of free riders; they pay to build the bus, they pay to fill it with fuel, and they pay to hire the driver. But pharmaceutical corporations still demand a prohibitive fare if those taxpayers wish to take a seat.

12

MEDICINE PATENTS ARE EXTENDED
TOO FAR AND TOO WIDE

The international standard for the length of patents on new medicines is twenty years. That standard was set by the 1994 Agreement on Trade-Related Aspects of Intellectual Property Rights, known as the TRIPS Agreement, which we learn more about in chapter 18. For essential medicines, that twenty-year monopoly guarantees two things: high prices for patent-holders and the resulting barriers to treatment for patients. But pharmaceutical corporations are rarely content with even a twenty-year monopoly on the medicines they sell, so they engage in a variety of tactics to extend that period.

From the perspective of for-profit corporations, the reasons for pursuing extensions are understandable: when a branded medicine goes off-patent, generic alternatives can come on the market, usually priced at a fraction of the branded version. At that point, the sales of the branded medicine can drop by as much as 90 percent or more.[1]

For some pharmaceutical corporations, that sales drop is the equivalent of falling off a financial cliff. For example, the allergy drug Claritin accounted for one-third of the revenues of Schering-Plough before it went off patent; in addition, Prozac once provided more than one-quarter of the revenues of Eli Lilly.[2] Delaying that huge financial hit by extending a patent for even a few months or years can mean hundreds of millions of dollars to a pharmaceutical company. When the corporation Celaphon achieved an extension of its monopoly on the sleep-disorder drug Provigil in 2006, the company CEO was barely able to contain his excitement: "We were able to get six more years of patent protection. That's $4 billion in sales that no one expected."[3]

So it is not surprising that pharmaceutical corporations are eager to hire what some industry observers call "floors full of lawyers" to pursue patent extensions. Here are some of the corporate tactics that are used to prolong monopoly patents—and the high medicine prices that go along with them: evergreening, data exclusivity, patent thickets and patent linkage, and buying off competitors.

Evergreening

Evergreening occurs when a new patent is granted for minor revisions or new uses of an already patented medicine, thus extending monopoly control past the original twenty-year period.[4] Evergreening is also sometimes referred to as secondary patenting. One study showed that secondary patents block generic competition on average more than six years, providing monopoly extensions that earn corporations—and cost patients—billions of dollars.[5]

Here is an example of how it works. In South Africa, the company Novartis obtained a patent in 1993 for the drug imatinib, a treatment for chronic myeloid leukemia that is marketed by the company under the name Gleevec. Before that South African patent was scheduled to expire in 2013, Novartis obtained two additional patents on the drug: one in 1997 for a new form of the compound and one in 2002 for the use of the drug to treat an HIV-related infection. The drug is now on patent in South Africa until 2022, twenty-nine years after the original patent was granted. In contrast, in India, where evergreening is blocked by its patent laws, there are no secondary patents on imatinib. The medicine is available in generic form, and costs 91 percent less than the South African version.[6]

The evergreening process is quite common, especially with drugs that are big sellers, even though this approach completely contradicts the self-promotion of the pharmaceutical industry as a force for innovation and new treatments.[7] The practice of evergreening, combined with the "me too" market-chasing focus of drug development, is the reason behind a startling fact: most new chemical entities patented by drug companies do not provide any new treatment value to patients. Researchers call that value therapeutic innovation, and precious few drugs offer it. One recent analysis estimated that 70 percent of newly marketed drugs offered no additional therapeutic value.[8] Similarly, a 2009 European Commission study found that 87 percent of the medicine patents recently granted or pending in the European Union countries were secondary patents, most likely in pursuit of evergreening.[9]

Although insulin was first patented in 1921, it is currently not available generically in the United States, setting the stage for the three manufacturers of insulin to raise their prices more than 160 percent in recent years. Costs for U.S. diabetes patients are six times higher than in other developed nations.[10] A contributing factor to the prohibitive pricing has been the numerous patents insulin manufacturers have obtained on changes made during the ninety-plus years since its original discovery. There is debate over the relative value of those patented improvements. "I don't think it takes a cynic such as myself to see most of these drugs are being developed to preserve patent protection," David Nathan, a Harvard Medical School professor, told the *Washington Post* in 2016. "The truth is they are marginally different, and the clinical benefits of them over the older drugs have been zero."[11] The U.S. publication *Business Insider* entitled a 2016 article about insulin pricing, "A 93-Year-Old Drug That Can Cost More Than A Mortgage Payment Tells Us Everything That's Wrong With American Healthcare."[12]

Data Exclusivity

Another patent-extending approach is for corporations to push for lengthy periods of data exclusivity to be inserted into national laws or international trade agreements. To understand data exclusivity, it helps to recognize that there are actually two separate processes that allow pharmaceutical companies to block competitors. The first is the patent system, which we have already discussed. The second is exclusivity, a period of time in addition to the usual twenty-year patent period during which no generic competition is allowed. Exclusivity is granted by a government agency—in the United States, it is the FDA.

The key form of exclusivity is known as data exclusivity. Here is how it works. When generic manufacturers apply for the right to distribute a drug, they need to show that the drug is safe and effective. An obvious way to demonstrate safety and efficacy is to cite test results on the identical and previously approved patented medicines. But data exclusivity blocks generic manufacturers from doing so.[13]

Without access to that test information, generic manufacturers are delayed in bringing their product to market, extending patent drug monopolies. The generic manufacturers may even have to repeat clinical trials on human subjects. That testing is not only expensive and time-consuming, it is unnecessary—because the drug has already been proven safe and effective—and thus ethically suspect.[14]

Data exclusivity periods are shorter than the twenty-year baseline length of patents. In the United States, most drugs have five years of data exclusivity, and biologics have twelve years. So why do drug companies still pursue them? The reason is that data exclusivity periods do not begin until the drug receives market approval, which may be several years after the company has obtained its patent. So if a biologic drug was patented ten years before it receives market approval, the corporation has only ten years in which to sell its drugs under a patent-protected monopoly. But a twelve-year data exclusivity decision gives the corporation an extra two years beyond the patent expiration to sell without generic competition.

One bizarre case from 2009 illustrates the difference between a patent and exclusivity. A pharmaceutical corporation conducted a one-week clinical trial on a medicine for gout that had been widely available since the nineteenth century. The corporation could not get a patent for the medicine, but the clinical trial allowed it to apply for and receive a period of data exclusivity. It used the exclusivity to force competitors out of the market, after which it raised the price of the medicine by 5,000 percent.[15]

The Obama administration has estimated that a five-year reduction in the twelve-year length of U.S. data exclusivity for biologic drugs would save federal health programs over $4 billion.[16] Think of what else that calculation means: the current data exclusivity rules now allow that extra $4 billion of taxpayer funds to be pulled in by monopoly drug pricing, along with a huge amount of direct costs shouldered by patients.

So it is no wonder that the pharmaceutical industry values data exclusivity so highly. As we learn in the conclusion to the book, the dogged pursuit by the industry of lengthy exclusivity for biologic drugs in the TPP became a sticking point in the debate over the trade deal.

Patent Thickets and Patent Linkage

Patent thickets, also known as patent clusters, are exactly what those nicely descriptive terms suggest they are: a dense pack of patents drafted by the "floors full of lawyers" to surround medicines that generate profits for pharmaceutical corporations. Would-be generic competitors must navigate that thicket of patents—one study found as many as 1,300 patents on a single drug—before they can offer their low-cost alternatives to patients.[17]

Patent linkage is the term for national laws or trade agreement terms that provide the platform for patent thickets to do their work. Linkage laws require generic competitors to prove that their product does not violate any of the hundreds or even thousands of patents protecting a monopoly drug. Even though many of those patents are quite suspect, linkage laws create a huge, time-consuming, and costly task list for would-be generic competitors to accomplish.

Together, thickets and linkage are quite effective at fending off generic competition. For example, the corporation AbbVie has a reported seventy-plus patents on its arthritis drug Humira, and these additional patents should add at least six years of monopoly protections on to the original Humira patent period. "Any company seeking to market a biosimilar version of Humira will have to contend with this extensive patent estate, which AbbVie intends to enforce vigorously," Richard A. Gonzalez, the AbbVie CEO, said in 2015.[18]

The motivation for these efforts is no mystery. Humira is the top-selling prescription drug in the world, and its $14 billion in sales in 2015 accounted for more than 60 percent of the total revenue of AbbVie.[19] Every day that AbbVie can extend its monopoly represents millions of dollars in revenue for the company.

AbbVie is far from alone in exploiting patent thickets. A 2010 study published in the *Northwestern Journal of Technology and Intellectual Property* examined multiple examples of the tactic and concluded, "The linkage regulation regime in particular has proven to be an excellent vehicle for firms to obtain extended legal protection on drugs at all stages of development, including drugs about to come off patent protection."[20] Economists call this activity by patent-holders rent-seeking, so named because it seeks to collect revenue without producing anything new or useful. Under rent-seeking, innovation takes a back seat to protecting monopolies. "[Pharmaceutical] companies today have found that the return on investment for legal tactics is a lot higher than the return for investment for R&D," said one health insurance executive.[21] Do not look for that statement to be repeated on any PhRMA public relations material anytime soon!

Buying Off Generic Competitors, AKA "Pay for Delay"

Patent thickets and patent linkage provide pharmaceutical corporations with significant leverage that allows them to engage in what one commentator called a "sleazy and blatantly self-serving" patent extension tactic: buying off would-be generic competitors.[22]

A company that wants to sell a generic version of a drug that is coming off its original patent faces a significant problem: before it can sell its product, it probably has to overcome costly, years-long, thicket-citing lawsuits filed by the deep-pocketed, highly motivated corporation that holds the patent(s). But there is another, less onerous option for the generic competitor, known as "pay for delay." The generic company can, instead, accept a large check from the patent-holding corporation in return for an agreement to delay its entry into the market.

There is a clear mutual incentive for such a deal. Because the generic company would sell the medicine at a sharply reduced price, its limited expected profits can be easily matched or exceeded by a big check from the patent-holding corporation. For the patent-holder, that check amount is still less than the company would lose by surrendering the monopoly that allows it to mark up the price tag of the drug to a level far above what the generic company would charge. Both companies win. The only loser is the patient, who is still forced to pay the monopoly price for the medicine she needs.

Remarkably, pay for delay is arguably legal in the United States, despite recent efforts by the Federal Trade Commission (FTC) to ban the practice as a violation of the antitrust laws.[23] The U.S. Congress has not been any help in that effort—remember the heavy lobbying and campaign expenditures by the pharmaceutical corporations?—and a 2013 U.S. Supreme Court decision did not fully clarify the issue.[24] Meanwhile, as Jon Leibowitz, former FTC chair, has characterized the current status quo, "Instead of competing to be first to come to market, generic companies compete to be first to get paid off."[25]

These industry tactics can get a bit difficult to keep track of, so it is important to remember why they matter: they are all corporate schemes whose aim is to prevent us from accessing generic medicines, which can be anywhere from 40 to 90 percent cheaper than the patent-protected medicines. So the impact of pay for delay, along with evergreening, packet thickets, and patent linkage, is enormous.[26] A 2012 study found that eliminating just evergreening in the United States could allow over one-third of currently patent-protected medicines to be immediately open to generic competition. Barring evergreening would also reduce by four or five years the delays in other patented drugs being open to competition.[27] As for pay-for-delay schemes, the FTC estimates they cost U.S. patients an extra $3.5 billion each year.[28]

Of course, for patients who cannot afford the cost of monopoly-protected medicines, whether they live in the United States or in other countries, patent extensions are not measured in dollars and cents. Their impact is felt in sickness, suffering, and even death.

13

PATENT PROTECTIONISM STUNTS THE DEVELOPMENT OF NEW MEDICINES

As we have seen, monopoly patent protections are defended by corporate medicine manufacturers on the grounds that patents are necessary to spur innovation.[1] The power of that argument is undeniable. We all want researchers to uncover new and better medicines that can improve our health and the health of our loved ones. And it is certainly logical to conclude that the rewards of a monopoly patent will create an incentive to invent something new.

But, as it turns out, both the history of innovation and recent trends in creative inventions show that patents do exactly the opposite. Patents do not, on the whole, trigger innovation in medicines. In fact, the evidence shows they actually discourage new discoveries and ideas. The incentive to innovate to receive a monopoly patent reward is certainly present, but the positive impact of that incentive is dwarfed by the negative effects that monopolies have on subsequent innovation. As economists Michele Boldrin and David Levine bluntly put it, "The case against patents can be summarized briefly: there is no empirical evidence that they serve to increase innovation and productivity. . . . (T)here is strong evidence, instead, that patents have many negative consequences."[2]

Why do patents actually hurt innovation? It is because patents are government-imposed zones of exclusivity, preventing the sharing of information that could lead to new discoveries.[3] Some scientists have been critical of patents on philosophical grounds, noting that science is built on the broad sharing of information that allows conclusions to be confirmed or rejected, and interim discoveries to be built on.[4] Economists who study the effects of patents have described them as "dead weight" on the process of innovation.[5] Others characterize them as "an unnecessary evil."[6]

In the field of medicines, we have already seen evidence of that dead weight piled on by patents. If researchers were not walled off from information about the medicines, they could take existing formulas and improve on them, or use them as the foundation on which to build new medicines altogether.[7] Instead, as we have seen (chapter 12), patent-holders use data exclusivity, patent thickets, and other tactics to block follow-up competitors.

Representatives of large pharmaceutical companies have admitted that even their own research is limited due to other companies holding patents on key molecules.[8] Patents create a burden on innovation in other fields as well. A survey by the Intellectual Property Owners Association showed that even its members from large corporations felt there was overpatenting in the current system.[9]

Economic analyses of patent and invention history tell us that the great majority of innovations have occurred outside the patent system and that countries without patent laws have produced more than their share of inventions, including inventive new medicines.[10] For example, Petra Moser, a New York University economics professor, studied the effects of compulsory licensing, in which the government overrides a patent and allows generic production. She found that these patent overrides opened up the field and encouraged innovation.[11]

Historical data have shown that the reverse is true as well: monopolies granted by patents have consistently discouraged innovation.[12] For example, the patenting of gene sequences in the Human Genome Project has been estimated to have slowed further innovation by 20 to 30 percent.[13] Three-quarters of biomedical researchers report that patents have hampered their access to materials and information needed for their research.[14] The U.S. Constitution provides Congress with the power to establish patents, but specifically with the purpose "to promote the progress of science and useful arts."[15] Especially in the case of essential medicines, that constitutional intent has been undermined by the current use of patents to stunt scientific progress, not promote it.

We do not need to look far for proof of the benefits of open access to information. There is recent dramatic evidence that removing the barriers to innovation created by intellectual property rules can be enormously valuable to the public. That evidence has been provided by the open-source software movement. Allowing multiple creative minds to improve and build on existing software has led to remarkable innovations in the fields of health care, education, and communication.[16] Most websites rely on open-source software, as do Google, Amazon, and Android smartphones, among many, many other products.[17] An analysis of the field shows that software engineers are demonstrably more efficient than they were before open source took hold.[18]

Medicine researchers have noticed this success and launched new initiatives to provide open sharing of research data on malaria, TB, and other neglected diseases, a model that deliberately rejects the corporate practice of secrecy in drug development.[19] As one researcher told the British medical journal the *Lancet* in 2016, "True open source should . . . unleash talents not already there; the enthusiasm of scientists with day jobs who love problem solving or doing altruistic work in their spare time; female scientists excluded from the workplace who can manipulate molecules on home computers, or even companies that undertake pro-bono work on open-source projects to impress potential clients."[20] Other researchers who studied the discovery of drugs that have the most impact have concluded that encouraging open-source development would be a much more effective public policy approach than continuing to throw patent monopoly benefits to pharmaceutical corporations.[21]

If knowledge about medicine was made as freely available to researchers as software code is to programmers, we can only imagine what new and important medicines could be discovered. For now, however, medicine patents—and the culture of profit, secrecy, and protectionism they represent—stand in the way.

14

GOVERNMENTS, NOT PRIVATE CORPORATIONS, DRIVE MEDICINE INNOVATION

We have already learned that the pharmaceutical industry investment in research and development is greatly exaggerated (chapter 6). We have also learned that the drugs the industry does develop are usually long on profit and short on treatment value and innovation (chapter 5). So, who is doing the research that actually leads to new and valuable medicines? You are. Or, at least, you are paying for it. Governments, using taxpayer dollars, have long been the most impactful supporters of the innovation that leads to the most important medicines.

The best estimates are that about 40 percent of medicine research and development costs are shouldered by governments and private philanthropy, not private corporations.[1] That number is much higher than pharmaceutical industry rhetoric would have us believe, but even that 40 percent figure vastly understates the key role played by governments. Government investments in medicine research are heavily weighted at the front end of the process, the basic research that is essential to identifying how a disease may be vulnerable to attack by medicines. The results of that basic research can provide the building blocks for many drug discoveries down the line.

That early-stage research is also time-consuming, expensive, and often quite frustrating. By virtue of its place in the research and development sequence, this research is several steps removed from a finished product that is ready for sale. All these factors make basic research an unappealing investment for a for-profit drug corporations. So these corporations turn to governments, especially the U.S. NIH, to handle this riskiest part of medicine research. The NIH annual budget for medical research is now over $32 billion per year, most of it spent supporting university-based research.[2]

No one knows the importance of this support better than the researchers themselves. In the early 1980s, the legendary biochemist Peter Berg attended an event at which he heard a venture capitalist extolling the financial investments of his sector in genetic engineering. Berg, one of 148 Nobel Prize winners who have received research funding from the NIH, could not help interrupting.[3] "Where were you guys in the '50's and '60's when all the funding had to be done in the basic science?" he asked. "Most of the discoveries that have fueled (the industry) were created back then. I can't imagine that, had there not been an NIH funding research, that there would be a biotech industry."[4]

For the most valuable medicines, governments play a particularly crucial role. While profit-seeking pharmaceutical corporations are searching for the next big-selling "me too" drug, the NIH and other government funders are leading the way in discovering the medicines that are innovative and important. Consider the origins of the medicines that the FDA identifies as the most valuable, those deserving "priority review" status. That designation means the medicines will provide "significant improvements in the safety or effectiveness of the treatment, diagnosis, or prevention of serious conditions."[5] A study of drugs receiving the priority review status from 1988 to 2005 showed that two-thirds of them traced their roots back to government-funded research.[6]

Another study went further back, looking at the twenty-one of the most important medicines discovered from 1965 to 1992. It turns out that fifteen of them relied on U.S. government-funded research.[7] Similar analyses of the origins of drugs that are considered transformative found that many were based on discoveries made by academic researchers using government funding, with the industry usually taking on a role only after these promising results were revealed.[8] Even that dynamic has shifted over the years, with U.S. law changes in 1980 (see chapter 15) spurring government-funded researchers to move increasingly into the applied-research stage of the drug-discovery process, especially for the most important medicines such as vaccines and medicines to treat cancer and infectious diseases.[9]

But even the impressive results of these studies understate the role of governments. The studies looked only at direct government research funding, which does not account for the significant indirect support given to the pharmaceutical industry for research by way of tax credits that can reach as high as 50 percent.[10] (I discuss in chapter 15 the role of government in subsidizing the industry by serving as the bulk, and often nondiscounted, purchaser of its products.) Once direct government support and generous tax breaks are added to the equation, some analysts calculate that private industry pays for only one-third of U.S. biomedical research—and much of that industry contribution is focused on drugs whose chief value is profit, not better health.[11]

There are many examples of lifesaving medicines that we rely on now that exist because of government research. The enormously valuable cancer drug pacilataxel was developed by research funded by the National Cancer Institute, a division of the NIH.[12] Government funding played the critical role in the breakthrough development of the antiretroviral medicine AZT and the highly effective leukemia drug imatinib.[13] The same is true for major mental health medicines and many vaccines.[14]

Most patients and taxpayers are not aware of the government parentage of these and other key medicines. The critical government role is obscured from view by U.S. laws pushed through by the pharmaceutical lobby (see chapter 15), which allow the patents for these and many other government-developed medicines to be handed over to private companies. The companies may do some end-stage development of the drug, a far less risky endeavor than the earlier research, and then sell the product at monopoly prices. As the economist Marianna Mazzucato points out, the United States "invests in the most uncertain stage of the business cycle and lets businesses hop on for the easier ride down the way."[15]

Sometimes, the companies are called out on their myth-making. In 1989, the CEO of the AZT patent-holding corporation Burroughs

Wellcome publicly boasted about the role of the company in the development of the drug. For the five researchers who coauthored the first publications identifying AZT as a treatment for AIDS, the corporate bragging was too much to bear. In a coauthored letter to the *New York Times,* they said the CEO's claim was "astonishing in both substance and tone." The researchers laid out how government support allowed the first synthesis of AZT to be performed, provided the first demonstration of its use on retroviruses, and was the foundation for every other critical stage of the development of the drug. "In a number of specific ways, government scientists made it possible to take a drug in the public domain and make it a practical reality as a new therapy for AIDS," they wrote. As for Burroughs Wellcome, the researchers said, the company was more of an impediment than a helper: "Indeed, one of the key obstacles to the development of AZT was that Burroughs Wellcome did not work with the live AIDS virus nor wish to receive samples from AIDS patients."[16]

It is worth pointing out that the critical role of government in supporting innovative research goes beyond the field of medicines. Most science historians agree that the three most influential technological developments of the twentieth century were the creation of the Internet, the discovery of the chemical structure of DNA, and the breakthroughs in nuclear energy. All were based on publicly funded research.[17] In fact, if we check under the hood at the engine driving many of the modern private-sector success stories, we will often find government-funded research. The Google search algorithm and the iPhone touch-screen and global positioning system (GPS) technology are all based on government research.[18] And as Paul Berg pointed out thirty years ago, the government was particularly critical in laying the foundation for modern biotechnology.

No less of a free market fan than Bill Gates, Microsoft founder, recently decided to take a close look at the record of government-sponsored innovation and came away impressed. "Since World War II, U.S.-government R&D has defined the state of the art in almost every area," Gates said in 2015. "The basic-science money is very well spent. The government has these 'Centers of Excellence.' They [the government] should have twice as many of those things, and those things should get about four times as much money as they do."[19]

15

TAXPAYERS AND PATIENTS PAY TWICE FOR PATENTED MEDICINES

I once heard a former member of the European Parliament provide a colorful explanation of the problem covered by this chapter. When it comes to medicines, he said, governments are like really dumb venture capitalists. Governments pay to develop a product but then hand over that product to an outside organization, declining to take an ownership interest. What is worse, governments later agree to purchase the product they developed and pay marked-up prices due to a monopoly they gave the organization they handed the product to.[1]

Of all the dumb medicines venture capitalists, none is dumber than the U.S. government. As we have seen in chapter 14, the U.S. government plays an indispensable role in funding the research that leads to the discovery of essential medicines. Until the 1980s, those taxpayer-financed breakthroughs were either owned by the federal agency that supported them or placed in the public domain, allowing patients to affordably access the medicines and researchers to build on the discoveries. But U.S. Senators

Birch Bayh (D-IN) and Robert Dole (R-KS), spurred on by pharmaceutical industry lobbyists, put a stop to that. They sponsored the Patents and Trademark Amendments Act, soon widely known as the Bayh-Dole Act, which allows universities and small companies that received federal research funding to claim patents for the discoveries that comes out of that research.[2]

Bayh-Dole went into effect in 1981, and universities and teaching hospitals wasted no time beating a path to the patent office. In the first five years under the new law, their human biology patent applications increased 300 percent.[3] Universities also quickly began forming partnerships with small biotech companies and, ultimately, with the large pharmaceutical corporations to conduct late-stage research and then market and distribute the medicines. Those corporations were happy to buy the exclusive rights to government-funded discoveries—and the monopoly pricing powers that went with them.[4]

Simply put, this is a give-away of government-created resources. U.S. taxpayers, in particular, pay twice for patented medicine: first to subsidize the research and then by way of the monopoly prices charged to government programs such as the Veterans Administration, Medicaid, and Medicare. As we see later (chapter 20), pharmaceutical industry lobbying has even succeeded in making it unlawful for the U.S. government to negotiate down the medicine prices paid by Medicare.

This scheme has inspired outrage from physicians, economists, and health activists. They call the corporate-government medicines arrangement a "parasitic relationship."[5] Alfred Engelberg, a noted intellectual property attorney, laid out the terms of this relationship in the publication *Health Affairs* in 2015:

> Federal law essentially socializes the cost of drug discovery while privatizing the profits since it does nothing to limit the prices that can be charged or the profits that can be earned from drugs discovered at public expense. . . . For decades, Congress has simply been transferring wealth from ordinary citizens to the pharmaceutical industry. While claiming to believe in free market capitalism, it has created a web of monopolies which cause the United States to pay the world's highest prices for drugs even though it is the largest purchaser.[6]

Examples of these taxpayer-to-corporation wealth transfers are plentiful. Consider these few:

- The corporation Genzyme charges as much as $350,000 per year, ten times its manufacturing cost, for a drug to treat the rare Gaucher disease. That price is often charged to government programs such as Medicaid, even though the medicine was developed by the NIH.[7]
- The corporation Amgen has billed Medicare for billions for the kidney disease drug Epogen, developed with taxpayer-supported research.[8]
- The story is the same for the chemotherapy drug pacilataxel, developed with government research and now sold back to government programs at monopoly prices by patent-holding BristolMyersSquibb, who has branded the drug Taxol.[9]
- NIH and U.S. Department of Defense funding helped develop the prostate cancer drug Xtandi, which is sold back to the federal government at over $100,000 per patient per year (a price that is two to four times that paid by patients in other countries), despite the fact that U.S. taxpayer dollars developed the drug.[10]
- Even the $1,000-per-pill hepatitis C medicines (see chapter 1) owe their existence to government research. In fact, the drugs were developed in part using funding from the U.S. Veterans Administration. Now, that same agency faces cuts in its services because of the need to pay a corporate monopoly markup for these medicines.[11]

The taxpayers-pay-twice arrangement is appalling, but it does provide an opening for the reform of our dysfunctional medicine system. As we see in chapters 20 and 21, there are many possible ways to make the medicine system better for both patients and taxpayers. At their core, these fixes would replace the waste and cost of the for-profit medicine model with approaches that rely on governments and nonprofits that answer to patients and taxpayers, not shareholders and corporate CEOs.

The good news is that the current government subsidy of the for-profit medicines model means there are plenty of funds to be shifted over to a system that will be both more effective and more fair. In his 2016 book, *Rigged: How Globalization and the Rules of the Modern Economy Were Structured to Make the Rich Richer*, the economist Dean Baker crunched the numbers and estimated the money that could be saved if U.S. health care systems could provide medicines without the artificial price markup imposed by monopoly patents. It turns out that the resulting savings could fund the replacement of all private industry research and development several times over, replacing that private research with more impactful and transparent studies while still leaving billions of dollars in remaining public benefits.[12]

Part IV

Trading Away Our Health

16

MEDICINES ARE A PUBLIC GOOD

Most of us define the term *public good* broadly. We use the term to refer to goods such as law enforcement, street lights, and mass transit, which are collectively provided and deliver shared benefits to all.[1] When economists describe public goods, they refer to these goods as being nonrivalrous and usually nonexcludable in their consumption.[2] We do not use those terms in everyday discussion, but their meaning is not that complicated. *Non-rivalrous* means that any one person can benefit from a good without reducing others' opportunity to benefit as well. My eating an apple means you cannot consume it, so that is a rivalrous good. But I can watch the same TV show as you without lessening your opportunity to enjoy it as well—that is nonrivalrous. *Nonexcludable* means what it sounds like: a person cannot be prevented from consuming the good in question. Clean air is a good that can be enjoyed by all without denying access to those who do not register or pay a fee. In contrast, access to a private swimming pool is an excludable good.

The classic example of a nonrivalrous, nonexcludable public good is a lighthouse: that one ship benefits from its warning does not subtract from the chances of any other ships enjoying a similar benefit, and there is no practical way of limiting the warnings from a lighthouse to a select few.

In terms of medicines, an individual pill is rivalrous—not everyone can consume that one pill—but the details of the formula for creating that pill are not. That formula is knowledge, and knowledge is a classic public good because it can be shared widely without penalty to the original owner. As Thomas Jefferson said, "He who receives an idea from me, receives instruction himself without lessening me; as he who lights his taper at mine, receives light without darkening me."[3]

But pharmaceutical corporations, with a big assist from the U.S. government, have responded to the nonrivalrous character of medicinal knowledge by cutting the wick off Jefferson's neighbor's candle. As we see in chapter 17, those corporations successfully pushed for international trade agreements that created the patent system. By prohibiting the use of patented medicine formulas by anyone except the patent-holder, that system artificially imposes exclusivity where none existed before. Economists call this process the transformation of a public good into a "club good."[4] The analogy is taking a public park and turning it into a gated, dues-required golf course.

Yet those legal maneuvers cannot obscure the fundamental nature of essential medicines: they are a public good. For example, access to medicines has public health implications, which create positive externalities, an economics term that means that one person's consumption of an essential medicine provides benefits beyond the direct consumer.[5] Vaccines provide the most obvious example of positive externalities because they prevent the recipient both from getting ill and also from spreading the disease to others. If a society vaccinates widely enough, the chain of disease transmission is broken, leading to a significant public good: widespread immunity. What could be more valuable to the public than the global distribution of the smallpox vaccine, which has led to the eradication of a disease that once infected 50 million people a year?[6]

Even medicines that are of less obvious population-wide benefit allow their recipients to better contribute to the social fabric and economic productivity of their communities. These medicines save costs for the broader society, too. When a diabetic takes insulin or a person with a risk for heart disease takes cholesterol-reducing medicine, he or she is more likely to make a positive contribution to the economy. Such people also lower their prospects of needing more extensive—and expensive—medical treatment, which is a cost often shared across multiple consumers and taxpayers.[7] The public good nature of medicines is further demonstrated by the potential negative externalities when people in need of medicines are deprived of them. The lack of access to medicine causes enormous social problems in terms of contagion and economy-depressing illnesses and premature deaths.[8]

Medicines are clearly a global good as well. The bubonic plague, cholera, influenza, HIV, and many other diseases have proven that the positive and negative externalities of access to medicine do not stop at national borders. Modern versions of medicines are most often developed in wealthy countries that are home to research-investing governments and corporations.[9] But those products are sometimes derived from plants and remedies that originated in low-income countries, which also provide the sites for many clinical drug trials.[10]

Among the public, medicines continue to be treated as a good quite distinct from consumer items such as cell phones and flat-screen TVs. That is because the unaffordability of a patent-protected consumer item does not invoke the moral challenge that comes with the impossibly high price tag placed on a lifesaving drug.[11] Millions of AIDS patients died in the 1990s and early 2000s because they could not pay for patented antiretroviral drugs, just as we have seen that millions die now due to lack of access to patented cancer medicines (chapter 4).

Tragedies such as these arouse the conscience of the global community. As a result, the human right to access essential medicines has found its way into international treaties and national constitutions.[12] Economists and philosophers have agreed that intellectual property rights should never trump the imperative to save the lives of human beings.[13] Faith-based organizations and civil society actors have advanced a moral claim for universal access to essential medicines.[14]

Researchers are well aware of the public-good nature of the products they are discovering. The creator of the first synthetic malaria vaccine donated the patent to the World Health Organization.[15] The inventors of insulin sold the patent to the University of Toronto for $1 each.[16] Jonas Salk declined to pursue a patent for the polio vaccine, saying the patent belonged to the people.[17] As Salk asked in 1952, "Could you patent the sun?"[18]

As Salk's comment suggests, medicines have proven to be a poor fit in the free market model. That model assumes the existence of well-informed consumers who exercise deliberate choices among competing products. But even thoroughly capitalistic societies have long recognized that the free market approach is not appropriate when the consumer is a sick person in urgent need of a remedy.[19] So, it is little wonder that, for nearly all of human history, societies and nations have treated medicines as a commonly held benefit. As we see later (chapter 17), until well past the middle of the twentieth century, few countries allowed individuals or companies to hold exclusive rights to produce medicines.[20]

Governments still take an extremely active, hands-on role in the medicines industry, creating the very opposite of a laissez faire market. Most industrialized governments tightly regulate the production and distribution of medicines, as well as actively promote vaccinations and encourage the safe use of other drugs.[21] Most of those countries, with the United States being a notable exception, also exert significant government control over the price of medicines.[22] Governments are both the leading funders of medicine research and the top purchasers of the end products of that research.[23]

Why do governments assume an activist role in the field of medicines? Because their citizens have demanded it. As we see in the conclusion to this book, grassroots-yet-global activism in the 1990s and 2000s gave voice to passionate outrage over the devastating human cost of limited access to patent-priced HIV/AIDS medicines. Demonstrators in the United States threw the ashes of AIDS victims on the lawn of the White House; global activists conducted mock trials charging pharmaceutical companies with genocide.[24]

These protests led to the dismantling of patent price barriers and, then, to massive government-funded programs. The same medicine that the patent-holding corporations once deemed too expensive for the global poor is now distributed to millions by the U.S. President's Emergency Plan for AIDS Relief (PEPFAR) and the Global Fund to Fight AIDS, TB and Malaria.[25]

But the HIV/AIDS treatment experience is not the norm. The U.S. government and pharmaceutical corporations have largely succeeded in their concerted effort to turn the public good of medicines into a for-profit commodity. In walling off access to medicine, corporations are following a disturbing historical precedent. Between the fifteenth and nineteenth centuries, the rich and the powerful in England managed to fence off commonly held land and transform it into private property.[26] The countryside was changed from a source of subsistence to a source of profit, and small farmers were relegated to wage laborers. The process is widely referred to as the enclosure movement, but in *Das Kapital*, Karl Marx described it by coining a new term: land-grabbing.[27] To Edward P. Thompson, a British historian, it was "a plain enough case of class robbery."[28]

Now, a similar enclosure movement is taking place.[29] This time, the fenced-off commodity is essential lifesaving medicines. Playing the role of modern-day lords of the manor are the pharmaceutical corporations, which have taken a good that was once considered off limits for private profiteering and turned it into an exclusive, expensive commodity. Instead of displacing small landholders, this particular enclosure movement causes suffering and death.

Medicine Patents Are Artificial, Recent, and Government-Created

As I discussed in chapter 16, medicines are clearly a public good. All of us understand in our hearts that it is profoundly wrong for a person to suffer because they cannot afford the price of a medicine that would comfort or even heal them. As we shall see later in this book, centuries of faith and moral traditions, more recently buttressed by human rights law, clearly support that view.

So why are essential medicines still unavailable to so many? To answer that question, we need to understand how corporations have recently written and promoted laws and trade agreements that elevate profits over people. The next few chapters may not be much fun to read, because they explain the many ways that these corporations have erected layers of complicated legal barriers blocking sick people from the medicine they need. But it is important to understand the path that led us to this shameful state in which people suffer needlessly. I promise that I will conclude this book by describing a very different path, one that leads us back to a place where medicine is treated as a public good. And I will share some stories of inspiring activists who are already blazing that trail for the rest of us.

When those activists, along with caregivers and researchers, argue today that lifesaving medicines and monopoly patents do not go together, they are actually following in the long-established traditions of intellectual property laws over many generations. Modern intellectual property law started when the governments of ancient Persia and Greece occasionally awarded exclusive rights to artists.[1] Monarchs in the Middle Ages granted some monopolies for purposes of political patronage or to block other territories from learning craft secrets.[2] "Letters patent," meaning open letters, were issued in fourteenth-century England to induce foreign crafts-men to relocate there.[3]

The first intellectual property law that systematically granted patents to inventors was adopted in Venice in 1474. Under that law, Venice care-fully preserved the right of the government to issue what are still known as "compulsory licenses." Under compulsory licenses, governments bypass patents when necessary and license non-patent-holders to manufacture the otherwise protected goods, with an accompanying responsibility to pay a royalty to the patent-holder.[4] Centuries later, compulsory licenses remain an important part of intellectual property law and are at the core of efforts to return medicines to their status as a public good.

Until well into the twentieth century, intellectual property rules did not exist in every nation, and they differed from one country to the next. Attempts to coordinate these varying global intellectual property rules led to the 1883 Paris Convention and the 1886 Berne Convention, and even-tually to the creation of the UN World Intellectual Property Organization in 1967.[5] But when nations signed on to those agreements, they retained the ability to determine the length of the patents and what products would be covered.[6] For many nations, that flexibility meant excluding medicines from patent protection. For example, the German patent law of 1877 labeled medicines "essential goods," along with food and chemicals, and prohibited any attempts to patent them.[7]

In the middle of the twentieth century, several post-colonial nations adopted laws that were similar to the German law.[8] The Indian pat-ent law extended only to the processes for creating medicines, not the chemical formulas of the drugs themselves.[9] (The United States, by con-trast, allows patents for both.[10]) So, the law in India opened the door for Indian pharmaceutical manufacturers to reverse-engineer patented drugs and then devise different, cheaper production methods.[11] This approach to medicine patent rights allowed India to become the site of a thriving generic drug industry, and the country became known as "the pharmacy of the developing world."[12]

The approach taken by India is not a new one. During the twentieth century, Brazil, Mexico, and other Central and South American countries also adopted limits on the patentability of medicines.[13] European countries such as Sweden and France did not grant pharmaceutical patents until the 1970s.[14] Spain refused to do so until 1992.[15] For decades, Switzerland had a constitutional prohibition on pharmaceutical patents.[16] In the mid-twentieth century, Italy was one of the world's leading producers of pharmaceuticals while prohibiting all drug patents until a Supreme Court ruling in 1978.[17]

Even when medicine patents were given, most laws included lots of exceptions. Many nations granted liberal access to compulsory licenses for patented drugs, meaning that generic manufacturers were free to make the drugs, as long as they paid a royalty to the patent-holders. For example, during the period between 1962 and 1992, Canada granted 613 licenses to import or manufacture pharmaceutical products.[18]

Over the course of human history, patent interests have been consistently limited in favor of ensuring access to medicines for those who needed them. As the UN special rapporteur in the field of cultural rights, Farida Shaheed, recently reminded the global community, there is no human right to patent protection. "The human rights perspective demands that patents do not extend so far as to interfere with individuals' dignity and well-being," Shaheed said in a 2015 report that explicitly cited concerns over patents limiting the accessibility of essential medicines. "Where patent rights and human rights are in conflict, human rights must prevail."[19]

By the late twentieth century, the scarcity of medicine patent protection, and the limitations and lack of uniform enforcement of medicine patents when they did exist, had become a real problem for pharmaceutical corporations. Over time, an industry that had once competed on the basis of manufacturing innovation and price had come to rely on the profits of products sold in the countries that enforced medicine patents.[20] Pfizer, for example, in the mid-twentieth century had a full 33 percent of its global sales attributable to just two patented drugs.[21] So, as extensively chronicled in Peter Drahos and John Braithwaite's 2002 book, *Information*

Feudalism: Who Owns the Knowledge Economy?, Pfizer executives decided to do something about it. They took the lead in an ambitious campaign to create a global system of intellectual property protection, a for-profit barrier between patients and the medicines they need.[22]

The first step in that effort was to counter the global norm that medicines were a public good. The pharmaceutical industry needed to establish a narrative that medicine compounds were property that could be owned by private companies and individuals, and that this private property should be protected by international law. An example of their efforts came in a high-profile July 1982 op-ed column in the *New York Times* by the chair of Pfizer International. That column, entitled "Stealing from the Mind," charged that U.S. inventions were being stolen by governments that did not protect patent rights. When governments outside the United States did not block the generic manufacturing of medicines, the pharmaceutical industry argued, they were indulging acts of piracy.[23]

The piracy allegation provided a vivid public relations image, but the industry executives realized that there was little in the way of binding international law to back up that position. So they pushed the U.S. government to make intellectual property protection a priority in all trade negotiations.[24]

It is worth pointing out that inserting monopoly patent rights into so-called free trade agreements creates an oxymoron. Patent exclusivity runs counter to the stated purpose of those agreements, the dismantling of barriers to global competition.[25] As Michele Boldrin and David Levine, economists, wrote in 2012, "Patents are very much akin to trade restrictions as they prevent the free entry of competitors in national markets, thereby reducing the growth of productive capacity and slowing down economic growth."[26] Another economist compared drug patents to a 10,000 percent tariff.[27]

But that contradiction did not stop the lobbying efforts by the pharmaceutical industry. And those efforts were quite successful, in large part because, then as now, the industry was reliably at the top of the U.S. lists in both lobbying expenditures and political campaign contributions. As U.S. Senator Richard J. Durbin (D-IL) said in 2002, "PhRMA, this lobby, has a death grip on Congress."[28] (Recall from chapter 15 that pharma lobbying had already achieved a coup when the Bayh-Dole Act of 1980 allowed private entities to claim monopoly patent rights on inventions discovered from government-funded research.) So it did not take long for the industry to find willing partners on Capitol Hill and in the White House.[29] Soon, the United States had adopted intellectual property protection as a litmus test for its trade partners.[30]

The role played by the U.S. government in this process was an essential one. As late as the 1980s, Drahos and Braithwaite write, a global treaty protecting patent rights was a business "pipe dream": "Why (would) more than one hundred nations that were large net importers of intellectual property rights sign an agreement that is so transparently against their interest, as well as being an economic and health disaster for them?"[31] As it turned out, the answer to that question was trade pressure exerted by the United States

That pressure was applied by way of carrots offered to patent-resistant countries—enhanced access to U.S. markets and some reductions in the subsidies of U.S. agricultural exports—while simultaneously brandishing some imposing sticks. In 1984, aggressive pharmaceutical-sector lobbying led to an amendment to the U.S. Trade Act that gave the president the authority to impose duties on, or withdraw trade benefits from, any nation that did not provide "adequate and effective" protection for U.S. intellectual property.[32]

The law was soon amended again to give the U.S. trade representative the power to put offending countries on what became known as a special 301 watch list, a designation dreaded by countries whose economies relied on trade with the United States[33] Soon, the two countries who resisted pharmaceutical patents most vigorously, India and Brazil, were placed in the more serious "priority" watch list and faced significant trade sanctions.[34]

Against this ominous backdrop, in 1986 the World Trade Organization (WTO) convened talks to create a global intellectual property agreement. At the time these talks began, more than forty of the ninety counties involved did not grant patents for pharmaceutical products, and others had adopted strict limits on them.[35] But the United States continued to wield big sticks: between 1985 and 1994, the U.S. trade representative brought special 301 actions dealing with intellectual property against Brazil, India, Argentina, Korea, Thailand, China, and Taiwan.[36] That pressure wore down even the once-firm resistance of countries such as Brazil and India, the latter of which was the final holdout.

By April 1994, the Agreement on Trade-Related Aspects of Intellectual Property Rights (TRIPS) was signed by 123 government ministers representing virtually the entire world community.[37] The deal finalized one of the foundational documents of the WTO, and it immediately became the most significant intellectual property agreement in history. As Edmund Pratt, the Pfizer CEO, later boasted, "Our combined strength enabled us to establish a global private sector-government network which laid the groundwork for what become TRIPS."[38]

TRIPS transformed an uneven worldwide patchwork of intellectual property law into a blanket of standards mandating protection for the holders of patents, copyrights, and trademarks. For patent-holders, that protection features at least twenty years of government-granted monopolies on their products, including medicines.[39] TRIPS also requires each nation to award intellectual property rights regardless of national origin, a boon for multinational pharmaceutical corporations and a death blow to their local manufacturing rivals.

As medicine activists would later lament, these corporations had essentially written the very regulations that were meant to govern them.[40] Big Pharma and the United States had succeeded in erecting a for-profit fence barring access to essential medicines.

18

THE UNITED STATES AND BIG PHARMA PLAY THE BULLY IN EXTENDING PATENTS

Unfortunately for sick people in low-income countries, the 1994 signing of the TRIPS Agreement did not signal an end to the efforts of the United States and pharmaceutical companies to put up a monopoly pay wall around essential medicines. TRIPS was a watershed moment for corporate patent rights, but from the pharmaceutical-company perspective, it was not quite perfect. TRIPS includes some concessions to the needs of low-income countries facing public health crises, including provisions that allow those countries to import generic medicines or permit the domestic manufacturing of generics when the public interest calls for access to less expensive medicines.[1] These terms are widely known as "TRIPS flexibilities." While the ink was still drying on the TRIPS Agreement, the United States and pharmaceutical corporations moved to block the use of those flexibilities.

In the late 1990s, when Brazil began to respond to its HIV/AIDS crisis and the unaffordability of patent-protected antiretroviral medicines by licensing the generic manufacturing of the drugs, the United States filed a complaint with the WTO.[2] When the South African Parliament responded to its own emergency by passing 1997 legislation to allow the importation of generic antiretroviral medicines, thirty-nine pharmaceutical corporations and a trade association sued the Nelson Mandela government to block the law.[3]

The U.S. Bill Clinton administration, whose relationship with the Pharmaceutical Research and Manufacturers of American (PhRMA) was so close that the brother of the president's chief-of-staff, John Podesta, served as a lobbyist for the industry, aggressively supported the lawsuit brought by the pharmaceutical companies against South Africa.[4] An official from the Office of the U.S. Trade Representative called the South African effort to obtain cheaper AIDS medicine "offensive," the administration placed South Africa on the trade watch list, and favorable tariff treatment for South African imports was denied.[5] Similar pressure from the United States forced Thailand to drop its own plans to allow the generic manufacturing of antiretrovirals.[6] Fortunately, as we see in the conclusion to this book, medicine activists in Brazil and South Africa, joined by a global coalition of allies, forced the U.S. government and the corporations to back down.

But the U.S. government and Big Pharma learned a lesson from those experiences: the fence TRIPS built around essential medicines had too many gates for their liking. So they embarked on a multidecade process of locking up those gates via what came to be known as TRIPS-Plus agreements. Article One of the TRIPS Agreement allows countries to "implement in their law more extensive (patent) protection than is required by this Agreement."[7] The United States has seized that part of TRIPS as an opportunity to push for stricter levels of medicine patent protections in its post-TRIPS trade agreements. The platforms for more stringent medicine patent protections were deals negotiated with just one other country, known as bilateral agreements, or regional trade agreements that included a limited number of countries.[8]

TRIPS-Plus deals used the same tried and true carrot-and-stick approach that had created TRIPS. Serving as the carrots were concessions in trade terms for agricultural products or textiles, which opened up the lucrative U.S. market to less wealthy nations. In bilateral agreements, the sticks can be particularly imposing: the withdrawal of trade relations altogether, or a cut-off in foreign assistance.[9] For example, Thailand did eventually decide to defy U.S. wishes and took steps to allow the domestic generic manufacturing of antiretroviral drugs, along with a much-needed heart medication. In response, the U.S. trade representative cited "indications of a weakening respect for patents" and placed Thailand on the same dreaded special 301 priority watch list that had brought so many other countries to heel during the TRIPS negotiations.[10]

Sometimes, the U.S. pro-Pharma pressure goes beyond mere trade sanctions. In 2016, the U.S. trade representative and a U.S. Senate staffer were accused of threatening Colombia with the loss of $450 million in promised U.S. funds for a national peace process if Colombia followed through with a proposal to use its TRIPS flexibilities to allow the generic manufacturing of a leukemia drug. The drug was patented by Novartis and priced at nearly twice the national income of Colombia, and the Colombian minister of health called efforts to sharply reduce that cost "a question of survival." The U.S. trade representative later denied directly threatening the loss of the peace funds, but advocates say that the message was clear enough. "We always assume that this kind of intervention is happening behind the scenes but rarely do you get the chance to see it up close," Andrew Goldman, an attorney for the medicine access group Knowledge Ecology International, told the Associated Press.[11]

The result of the TRIPS-Plus pressure has been a number of trade agreements that cement the monopoly rights of medicine patent-holders even more firmly than TRIPS does. TRIPS-Plus agreements include broader availability for the evergreening of patents, extending patents beyond the twenty-year TRIPS minimum; blocking importation of generics; and limiting the ability of countries to license domestic generic manufacturing.[12] The impact of these concessions may even extend beyond those countries that have bowed to U.S. pressure. A clause in TRIPS, usually referred to as the most-favored-nation provision, requires that an advantage granted to one country be granted to all. That promise sets the stage for the U.S.-forced TRIPS-Plus terms to become the de facto global standards.[13]

The bullying by United States and Big Pharma on patent rights is enormously harmful to people in developing countries. Consider the problem in South Africa, where HIV-positive patients are at risk because patented medicines are often out of stock. This presents a particularly dangerous situation with HIV/AIDS medications because when a patient who misses the scheduled doses, the virus can develop a resistance to the effects of the medicine. "The problem is very big, because it's life and death," says Thandi Shabangu, a South African HIV patient who has faced stock-outs of her medicine. "If you don't drink your Alluvia (lopinavir/ritonavir), you are going to resist."[14]

These are indeed life and death problems, and there is a clear solution to them. There should be no restrictions on essential medicines being manufactured in the countries where they are needed. Countries such as India, Brazil, Mexico, and China have proven manufacturing capacities and the ability to make and sell medicines cheaply, which would also boost their local economies with much-needed jobs and incomes.[15] The Indian pharmaceutical sector employs 4.5 million people and reliably produces high-quality medicines at a fraction of the cost of the patented versions.[16] Other low- to middle-income countries stand ready and eager to follow the lead of India.[17]

But that is not happening. Instead, most of the world's drug production takes place in wealthy countries.[18] And aggressive TRIPS-Plus enforcement of patent monopolies by the U.S. government and the pharmaceutical industry will keep it that way. Health activists such as Médecins Sans Frontières/Doctors Without Borders (MSF) have documented that the patent monopolies are blocking new manufacturers from entering the vaccines markets.[19] These monopolies are stopping the in-country production of much-needed generic HIV/AIDS and cancer medicines, too.[20] Now, the United States and the pharmaceutical industry are using trade pressure to try to also squeeze India out of the low-cost medicine business.[21]

People in low-income countries need medicines, and they need jobs, too. Too often, they get neither, thanks to wealthy corporations that insist that the only medicines that are allowed to be manufactured are their monopoly-protected products, which are then priced out of the range of affordability. Those corporations have ascended to dizzying financial heights, only to use patent enforcement to kick away the ladder before poor countries can do any climbing of their own.

The promotion by the U.S. government of medicine patent protection overseas is not always matched by its respect for patent rights in our own country, at least when a public health crisis appears. That hypocrisy became apparent one week after the devastating attacks of September 11, 2001, when the United States was confronted with a new threat:

the purposeful spread of the deadly infectious disease anthrax. Envelopes containing anthrax spores, postmarked September 18, 2001, were mailed to major U.S.-based media outlets. Two more infected envelopes, these post-marked October 9, 2011, were mailed to two U.S. senators. Twenty-two people were infected with anthrax due to the mailings, and five died.[22]

The only approved oral treatment for anthrax was the antibiotic ciprofloxacin, patented and marketed in the United States by Bayer Corporation under the name Cipro. This presented a problem: there was a limited supply of Cipro in the United States, and the price was thirty times higher than in nations where generic versions were available.[23] The response by the U.S. government was swift. Tommy Thompson, the secretary of the U.S. Department of Health and Human Services, demanded that Bayer significantly discount the price of Cipro. If Bayer failed to do so, Thompson vowed to seek congressional approval to obtain a generic version of the medicine. "The price is the question, not the supply," Thompson told a congressional committee in October 2001.[24] After Thompson's testimony, the chair of that committee publicly stated that any request to bypass the Bayer patent would probably be approved by Congress.[25] But that proved to be unnecessary. Bayer got the message and responded by cutting its Cipro price in half and pledging to provide 100 million tablets.[26]

This U.S. response was revealing. When it faced its own perceived public health crisis, the level of U.S. respect for the sanctity of medicine patents proved to be quite different from the stance it assumed in trade negotiations with lower-income countries. The contrast did not go unnoticed. "Even where there is clear evidence of a public health emergency, such as the HIV crisis in Africa and many parts of Asia, the U.S. government has used its might to limit these countries' options to provide affordable drugs," wrote the editors of the respected British medical journal *The Lancet* in November 2001. As *The Lancet* editors pointed out, the United States had recently lodged complaints to the WTO against Brazil and had supported the lawsuit by the pharmaceutical industry to block access to generic HIV/AIDS medicine in South Africa. "[P]ublic health needs may have to override trade profits," the editors wrote. "The U.S. government should apply the same standards abroad as at home."[27] Advocates for access to generic HIV medicines quickly seized the opportunity to point out U.S. hypocrisy on the issue.[28]

It turns out that the U.S. threat to break the Cipro patent was not a new approach. Instead, it was just the latest in a long line of examples of the United States overriding intellectual property rights when it suits its domestic interests, all while insisting on the strict enforcement of those rights by other nations. In the late eighteenth and early nineteenth centuries, the United States did not allow foreigners to file for patents at all, and the United States dragged its feet for over a century before finally signing the 1886 Berne Copyright Convention.[29] The U.S. Capitol building is literally built on a foundation of patent infringement: the concrete on the Capitol grounds was laid, without permission, in a manner that had been previously patented by one John J. Schillinger. The U.S. Court of Claims threw out Schillinger's patent infringement suit, ruling that the U.S. government had immunity from such claims.[30]

The most famous case of the United States conveniently bypassing patent rights involved a couple of stubborn American icons, a future president, and the demands of war. After their breakthrough discoveries in the invention of the airplane, Orville and Wilbur Wright proved to be as tenacious in defending their patent rights as they had been in pursuing motorized flight. In 1906, they obtained a patent for their method of flight control. For years afterward, the Wrights fiercely defended it, both in courts of law and in the court of public opinion. Wilbur Wright said in 1910, "It is our view that morally the world owes its almost universal use of our system of lateral control to us. It is also our opinion that legally it owes it to us."[31]

Together, the Wright Company and its rival, the Curtiss Company, held the major U.S. patents on airplane technology. They guarded their monopolies so jealously that the United States had fallen far behind Europe in the manufacture of planes. By 1917, as the United States was on the eve of entering into World War I, this was considered to be a national security problem.[32] In response, an ambitious young assistant secretary of the navy, Franklin D. Roosevelt, convened a committee that strong-armed the Wright and Curtiss companies into joining a "patent pool" called the Manufacturers Aircraft Association. Members of that pool were obligated to license their patent rights to other manufacturers in return for royalties.[33]

By 1949, the U.S. Congress had granted official permission to bypass patents on a grand scale. For example, 29 U.S. Code section 1498 allows the U.S. government, or anyone it authorizes, to manufacture a patented good or use a copyright without permission.[34] This provides a broad platform for issuing compulsory licenses, under which patent-holders are entitled to compensation for use of their products but cannot halt the manufacture of the items they have patented.

In this way, U.S. law opens wide the door to ignoring patent rights, and the government has quite often strolled right through. Following in the Wright-Roosevelt tradition, the United States has issued multiple compulsory licenses for patents to military technologies such as satellites, camouflage screens, and protective eyewear; it has also issued compulsory licenses for advances in energy technology and methods to reduce air pollution.[35]

Often, compulsory licenses have been the remedy of choice in resolving U.S. antitrust lawsuits, including the blunting of patents for the manufacture of truck parts, plastics, personal computers, corn seeds, microprocessors, animal vaccines, and gasoline.[36] The same U.S. trade representative who so vigorously pushed the extension of medicine patents in the proposed Trans-Pacific Partnership Agreement had also advocated that Apple be allowed to infringe on the smartphone patent rights of Samsung Electronics. The trade representative supported the breaking of the Samsung patent, he said, because the enforcement of the patent could be against the interests of U.S. consumers.[37]

The 2001 U.S. threat to override the Bayer Cipro patent was not the first time that the U.S. government determined that access to medicine and other health care technologies was more important than patent rights. In the late 1950s and early 1960s, the U.S. military repeatedly ignored the Pfizer U.S. patent for the antibiotic tetracycline; the military simply ordered a generic version for less than half the price from a manufacturer in Italy, where medicine patents were not enforced.[38] In 2004, the U.S. government threatened Abbott Laboratories with an override of its patent for the HIV/AIDS drug ritonavir. Like Bayer did when faced with the Cipro threat, Abbott got the message, and dropped its price 80 percent for patients in federally funded programs.[39] Antitrust litigation and threats of a government patent override have led to compulsory licenses being issued for stem cells, laser eye surgery, gene therapy, ultrasound imaging catheters, and the irritable bowel syndrome drug dicyclomine.[40] In a single five-year period, from 2006 to 2011, U.S. courts issued six different compulsory licenses for medical technologies.[41]

The U.S. President's Emergency Plan for AIDS Relief (PEPFAR) is reported to be the world's leading consumer of generic medicines manufactured under compulsory licenses.[42] In 2010, the U.S. Affordable Care Act included a mechanism for compulsory licenses to ensure U.S. access to patented biologic drugs.[43] The double standard is quite clear: for the U.S. government, the strict enforcement of health and medicine patents is a policy that poor nations must adhere to or face the consequences, but when enforcing those rules is not convenient in the United States itself, the need for enforcement seems to fade away.

We have discussed how the United States and pharmaceutical corporations achieved the piece-by-piece TRIPS-Plus erosion of the TRIPS flexibilities, the protections for affordable medicines included in TRIPS. But those setbacks paled in comparison to the potential sweeping impact of what was designed to be the most ambitious proposed TRIPS-Plus agreement of them all: the Trans-Pacific Partnership Agreement (TPP). At the time of this writing, the TPP has been put on indefinite hold, with U.S. President Donald Trump formally withdrawing the United States from the agreement.[44] (I discuss in the conclusion to this book the role that spirited activism in support of access to medicines played in the demise of the TPP.) But Trump's action was immediately followed by discussion of a partial revival of the TPP, or creation of a similar "son of TPP" pact.[45] So it is important to understand the dangerous TPP terms that are likely to find their way into future proposals, including a possible NAFTA renegotiation.

The intellectual property section of the TPP included the same "TRIPS-Plus" medicine patent–extending terms we have discussed earlier: evergreening of patents by allowing patent extensions for minor changes in existing medicines, investor-state dispute systems that allow corporations to force a government into arbitration over decisions that harm their interests (including refusals to grant or extend patents), and patent-linkage terms that provide a platform for litigation by corporate patent-holders.[46] All have the effect of delaying generic medicines from being available for patients in a country's market.

We know from previous TRIPS-Plus agreements the deadly impact of those medicine barriers. The intellectual property rules of the Central American Free Trade Agreement (CAFTA) when applied in Guatemala increased some medicine prices by 846 percent and blocked some generic drugs from entering the market.[47] The U.S.-Jordan free trade agreement caused a 20 percent increase in medicine prices and forced the Ministry of Health to spend a quarter of its budget on medicine. After that agreement went into effect, the prices of medicines in Jordan rose up to 800 percent higher than in neighboring Egypt.[48] After Morocco signed a patent-protecting 2006 trade agreement with the United States, spending on drugs there quickly doubled.[49] So it was not surprising when a study of the likely effect of TPP in Vietnam projected that the agreement would cause tens of thousands of HIV-positive Vietnamese patients to go without lifesaving treatment.[50]

But the TPP draft even went beyond the previous TRIPS-Plus agreements by including a new insistence on limiting access to affordable versions of biologic medicines. *Biologics* are treatments that are derived from a genetically-engineered, nonplant biological source—a human, an animal, or a microorganism. These medicines are usually much larger and more structurally complex than traditional small-molecule drugs.[51] Examples of biologics include vaccines, gene therapies, and many cancer drugs.[52]

Biologics play an important and growing role in medical treatment, but the patented versions of biologics dugs are often enormously expensive. For example, the breast cancer biologic drug trastuzumab, marketed by Roche as Herceptin, can cost as high as $70,000 for a course of treatment.[53] The biologic rheumatoid arthritis drug Remicade can cost $2,500 per injection.[54]

Because the costs of biologics is often so high, access to "biosimilars," more affordable generic-type alternatives, is critically important. But the TPP aimed to delay access to biosimilars by adding to patent protection the additional monopoly-protecting mechanism known as data exclusivity.[55] As I have previously discussed (chapter 12), data exclusivity means that the companies producing the nonpatented alternatives, in this case biosimilars, are blocked from accessing the testing data they need to get approval to sell their drug.

For biologics, TPP called for between five and eight years of data exclusivity.[56] Because testing is complicated and expensive, and there are ethical issues involved in conducting unnecessary testing, it is unlikely that biosimilar-producing companies will replicate the data for the biologics through their own testing. Instead, they will probably just wait out the data-exclusivity period before offering patients their less expensive alternative.[57]

The impact of this TPP barrier to biosimilars would have been enormous. Many important new medicines are biologics, especially cancer medicines, and patent-protected prices will place them out of the reach of patients in many low-to-middle-income nations.[58] Peru, Vietnam, Malaysia, and Mexico, which were all set to join as parties to the TPP, currently have no monopoly protection on data for biologics. "Now they'll have to wait at least five years before allowing cheaper biosimilars onto the market," said Judit Rius Sanjuan from MSF, when the deal looked to be moving forward. "It's a loss for people in developing countries. They'll face higher prices for longer periods of time, and there are many products we need that are biologics."[59]

In assessing the overall TPP damage to access to medicines, MSF said the deal promised to be the worst trade agreement in history.[60] As Zahara Heckscher, a breast cancer survivor, activist, and founder of CancerFAM, said, "Try telling a woman with breast cancer in Vietnam, where annual per capita income is under $2,000, that she has to pay $100,000 a year for the medicine that would save her life."[61]

The TPP was explicitly designed to be a template for future trade agreements.[62] So it's medicine-barring provisions are likely to be pursued again, putting millions at risk. All who are concerned about access to medicines must be on watch to prevent future trade agreements from wreaking the same kind of damage the TPP was slated to cause.

Pharma-Pushed Trade Agreements Steal the Power of Democratically Elected Governments

"Corporations are more powerful than governments." You may have heard this claim before, and you may have thought that it contains more than a little hyperbole. But in recent years, international trade agreements have indeed given multinational corporations special rights that provide them with the upper hand over democratically elected governments. Corporations can force these governments to pay billions of dollars in penalties simply for enforcing laws and policies that reduce corporate profits, even when those laws are in the best interests of their citizens. As you probably have guessed, that includes national laws that are designed to increase access to medicines. Even worse, those trade agreements are preventing governments from pursuing commonsense policies in the first place, simply because they fear corporate retribution. As some trade experts put it, we are living in a "Wild West" era where there are precious few limits on corporate power, including the power of the pharmaceutical industry.[1]

This corporations-trumping-governments dynamic is created by a provision of the trade agreements that requires countries to agree to investor-state dispute settlement (ISDS) systems. ISDS provisions allow corporations,

including pharmaceutical corporations, to force a treaty-signing government into binding private arbitration over government decisions that are
alleged to harm the corporation.[2] Specifically, if a corporation makes a
trade-agreement-inspired "reasonable investment-backed decision" and
the host government adopts a policy that harms that investment, the
government—and its taxpayers—has to pay the corporation.[3]

ISDS terms have been written into every trade deal the United States
has entered into over the past thirty years and into over 3,000 trade agreements worldwide.[4] Up until early 2017, two major trade agreements were
being hammered out: the Trans-Pacific Partnership Agreement (TPP) (see
chapter 18) and the Transatlantic Trade and International Partnership, a
proposed agreement between the United States and the European Union.
The TPP terms included ISDS provisions, and the United States is pushing hard for the inclusion of ISDS in any agreement with the European
Union. The watchdog organization Public Citizen has counted nearly
85,000 corporations that could have invoked ISDS powers under these
two agreements.[5]

The intent of the ISDS system is to bypass national courts and replace
them with a special process tilted in favor of the corporations. Here is
how that process works. ISDS claims are heard by a three-person panel
made up of attorneys, some of whom may actually represent corporations in their private practices.[6] In addition, the attorneys who have
been appointed to ISDS panels have incentives to increase their fees by
allowing cases to linger for years—the minimum fee for these ISDS panel
lawyer-arbitrators is $3,000 per day—and to pad their caseload by issu-
ing decisions that encourage more corporations to file ISDS challenges.[7]
There is no appeal of an ISDS decision. The most-used ISDS forum is part
of the World Bank, whose president has always been the candidate chosen
by the United States. Perhaps not surprisingly, the United States has never
lost an ISDS case.[8]

But most countries, especially less wealthy and less powerful countries,
cannot count on that kind of advantage when facing an ISDS challenge.
ISDS tribunals have already ordered countries to pay over $3 billion in
compensation to corporations.[9] That number is destined to go much
higher; beginning in 2011, corporations filed ISDS claims at the rate of
more than fifty per year, and nearly $40 billion in claims are pending.[10]

These claims directly challenge decisions made by governments that aim to elevate the health and well-being of the public over the profits of corporations. Tobacco companies have hauled the governments of Australia and Uruguay into ISDS proceedings when those countries tried to require cigarette warning labels, and they have threatened Canada with the same process.[11] Corporations have challenged efforts by Germany to curb corporate waste dumping into its rivers and to phase out nuclear power plants.[12] A Canadian province faces an ISDS challenge for imposing a limitation on the environmentally damaging practice of fracking, Mexico was forced into ISDS over its efforts to tax beverages using high fructose corn syrup, and an Ecuadoran court ruling was challenged using ISDS after it ordered corporate payment for the toxic contamination of the Amazon.[13] Although international law clearly dictates that human rights occupy a significantly higher status than intellectual property or other corporate rights, the often vague and ineffective accountability system for human rights violations pales in comparison to the specific and well-designed process for enforcing corporate interests.[14]

So far, U.S. taxpayers have been spared successful ISDS rulings, in part because U.S. policies are already among the most pro-corporate in the world. But the U.S. luck may soon run out. After President Barack Obama decided in 2015 not to pursue the Keystone XL oil pipeline due to environmental and cost considerations, the TransCanada Corporation invoked the ISDS terms of the North American Free Trade Agreement (NAFTA) and demanded a $15 billion payment to compensate for its investment in the proposed pipeline.[15]

More corporate claims are likely to follow. The Nobel Prize-winning economist Joseph Stiglitz explained the potential impact of ISDS in the context of recent U.S. history:

> Imagine what would have happened if these provisions had been in place when the lethal effects of asbestos were discovered. Rather than shutting down manufacturers and forcing them to compensate those who had been harmed, under ISDS, governments would have had to pay the manufacturers not to kill their citizens. Taxpayers would have been hit twice—first to pay for the health damage caused by asbestos, and then to compensate manufacturers for their lost profits when the government stepped in to regulate a dangerous product.[16]

Even U.S. Supreme Court decisions against a corporation could land the United States in an ISDS hearing room. As the law professor Brook Baker has written, it is easy to imagine how a Supreme Court ruling such as the 2013 decision that blocked the patenting of human genes could trigger a multibillion-dollar complaint from a foreign biotech firm that was counting on those patent profits.[17]

The idea of ISDS being used to block access to affordable medicines is not just a hypothetical exercise, as the pharmaceutical corporation Eli Lilly has proven. In 2009 and 2011, Canadian courts invalidated the Eli Lilly monopoly patents on two drugs, the attention-deficit hyperactivity disorder medicine Strattera and the psychiatric medicine Zyprexa.[18] The courts ruled that the drugs did not provide the therapeutic benefits the company had promised in its patent applications. Eli Lilly appealed these decisions to the highest levels of the Canadian court system and lost all of its challenges. For individuals and domestic corporations, these rulings would have meant the end of the line. But, thanks to the ISDS provision in NAFTA, a multinational corporation such as Eli Lilly is not limited by decisions handed down by the courts of a sovereign nation. Arguing that the corporation had a right to expect that Canada would not impose any medicine patent standards that were stricter than the most lenient standards in other nations, Eli Lilly filed a $500 million complaint under ISDS.[19]

In March 2017, Lilly's claim was denied. But other corporate ISDS challenges of medicine patent decisions have caused widespread alarm among health activists, and they shared their concerns with U.S. and Australian government representatives while those representatives negotiated the secret terms of TPP. In response, those country trade representatives promised that the ISDS provisions in the TPP would not apply to government decisions on intellectual property decisions such as medicine patents. Nevertheless, when the specifics of the TPPA were finally unveiled, they did allow corporations to use ISDS to challenge government patent decisions.[20]

The surprisingly wide scope of ISDS in TPP increased the global push-back against these enormous corporate privileges. The governments of South Africa and Indonesia are terminating their ISDS agreements, and the European Commission president and the German government are objecting to ISDS provisions being placed in future trade deals.[21] Even in the United States, whose officials lead the way in demanding ISDS be included in trade agreements, opposition is growing. Protests against the ISDS expansion of corporate power have been lodged by access-to-medicine activists, environmental and labor activists, state and federal lawmakers, and even conservative libertarian and Tea Party groups.[22]

In a June, 2015 statement, a group of UN experts that included the special rapporteur on the right of everyone to the highest attainable standard of health made it clear that ISDS provisions directly interfere with the ability of states ability to regulate in the public interest. The UN experts also pointed out that ISDS systems have a "chilling effect" that causes governments to be reluctant to adopt policies, including greater access to generic medicines, that may trigger an aggressive corporate response.[23] There is plenty of evidence that this chilling effect is quite real. For example, after the tobacco industry forced Australia and Uruguay into ISDS proceedings, both New Zealand and Canada backed away from mandating warnings on cigarette packages.[24]

ISDS rulings are made by arbitrators who are completely unaccountable to any voters, undermining both the national courts and the decisions of elected officials.[25] Consider the problems that would arise if the U.S. Congress ever decided to tighten up medicine patent requirements or reduce the length of medicine monopolies. A decision such as that would certainly be in the best interest of U.S. patients and taxpayers, but it would probably trigger multibillion-dollar ISDS challenges by foreign corporations with headquarters in countries that are parties to trade agreements with the United States As a result, the criticism of the ISDS, especially in the areas of health and environmental regulations, often centers on how ISDS "limits the policy space" for governments.[26]

That phrase—limits the policy space—is certainly correct. But it sounds a little too genteel to me. It would be more accurate to say that, when democratically elected governments make decisions that prioritize the health and well-being of their citizens, ISDS provides the vehicle for multinational corporations to bulldoze right over those decisions.

Part V

A Better Remedy

CURRENT LAW PROVIDES OPPORTUNITIES FOR AFFORDABLE GENERIC MEDICINES

The modern medicine system is clearly in desperate need of a major overhaul. But there is good news, too: not only are there big improvements that can happen if we change our corporate-influenced laws—improvements I discuss in chapter 21—there are significant improvements that can be made to our medicines system even without changing existing law.[1]

In chapter 17, we have seen that the TRIPS Agreement, which serves as the foundation of global medicine law, includes flexibilities such as the ability for governments to import generic medicines, a process commonly referred to as "parallel importation." TRIPS also allows governments to issue compulsory licenses, which permit the manufacturing of generic medicines in their countries. As far back as 1998, just four years after TRIPS was signed, James Love, a longtime medicine access advocate, argued that these flexibilities provided great opportunities. "The problem for developing countries is not whether compulsory licensing is legal, because it clearly is legal," Love said. "It's the political problem of whether they will face sanctions from the U.S. government for doing things they have the legal right to do but which the U.S. government does not like."[2]

Not too long after Love made that statement, global HIV/AIDS treat-ment advocates, helped along by the well-timed display of U.S. hypocrisy in medicine access in the response to the anthrax crisis after September 11, 2001, were able to open up the opportunities that Love described. As members of the World Trade Organization (WTO) prepared to gather for a meeting in Doha, Qatar, in November 2001, medicine activists were fresh from their success in shaming the United States and pharmaceutical corporations for walling off access to antiretroviral HIV/AIDS medicines (a campaign I discuss in the conclusion to this book). That same autumn, as we have seen in chapter 18, the United States had shown its own will-ingness to issue compulsory licenses in response to the perceived need for the patented medicine ciprofloxacin to counteract anthrax poisoning. When U.S. trade representatives sat at the negotiating table in Doha a few weeks later, they were in an unusually weak position from which to assert their characteristic argument that other nations should avoid the use of compulsory licenses.

That U.S. weakness helped lead to the WTO "Doha Declaration on the TRIPS Agreement and Public Health," which explicitly underscores the TRIPS flexibilities that allow medicine patents to be bypassed when public health needs call for it. In so doing, the WTO made it clear that current law elevates access to medicines and national autonomy above corporate patent rights: "We affirm that the [TRIPS] Agreement can and should be interpreted and implemented in such a manner supportive of WTO members' right to protect public health and, in particular, to promote access to medicines for all. . . . Each member has the right to grant com-pulsory licenses and the freedom to determine the grounds upon which such licenses are granted."[3]

This was an important statement. The Doha Declaration very clearly refuted a common misconception about TRIPS by stating in no uncer-tain terms that the freedom to issue compulsory licenses is not limited to times of emergency or crisis.[4] Doha also exempted the least-developed country members of the WTO from implementing pharmaceutical patent protection until January 2016, an exemption recently extended to 2032.[5] These decisions had real impact. In the years after Doha, the reaffirmed TRIPS flexibilities provided the platform for over fifty nations to produce or import generic HIV/AIDS medications. These measures saved millions of lives.[6]

The compulsory licensing and parallel importation flexibilities under TRIPS hold the potential for public health needs to be met while still providing patent-holders with profits. Compulsory licenses require that royalties be paid to the patent-holders but usually in the range of 4–6 percent, which is a far cry from the monopoly mark-ups that can be hundreds of times the cost of manufacturing the medicine.[7] Shamnad Basheer, an Indian legal scholar and a professor at West Bengal National University of Juridical Sciences, predicted that compulsory licenses will be on the rise globally because they represent a "middle path" between the overprotection of patents and the elimination of patents altogether.[8]

But, to date, the widespread use of compulsory licenses has not reached beyond the HIV/AIDS realm. For example, despite the crying need for more affordable cancer medicines, India and Thailand are the only nations that have issued compulsory licenses for cancer drugs.[9] Arguably, compulsory licenses are even more critical in the cancer arena than for HIV/AIDS because biosimilar drugs, the generic equivalent to the biologic medicines that have a growing presence in cancer treatment, are expensive to develop. Manufacturers may be reluctant to invest in developing biosimilars without first knowing that a compulsory license will guarantee that they will not face resistance from patent-holders.[10]

The global reluctance to employ TRIPS flexibilities to pursue generic medicines beyond HIV/AIDS medicines is no accident: the United States rebounded from its momentarily chastened post-anthrax state in 2001 to vigorously resume its practice of TRIPS-Plus bullying of countries such as Thailand, South Africa, and India, which dared to consider measures to reduce medicine costs. As a result, most low- and middle-income nations have avoided exercising their compulsory license rights beyond HIV/AIDS, despite similar needs in areas such as cancer. The South African campaign called Fix the Patent Laws is one of several efforts urging those governments to resist trade pressure and embrace the medicine-access flexibilities allowed them under TRIPS.[11]

Similar to these international laws, national laws in the United States provide a clear opportunity for the government to respond to problematic price mark-ups by monopoly medicine patent-holders. I have discussed (chapter 15) the problems caused by the Bayh-Dole Act of 1980, which allows government-funded discoveries to be patented and exploited by private corporations. But Bayh-Dole does provide taxpayers with a couple of escape hatches if the patent give-away proves problematic. The law allows any U.S. government agency that helped fund the development of a patented medicine—a quite common scenario, as we have learned in chapter 14—to retain the ability to license the generic manufacture of the patented medicine.

There are two ways that this escape hatch can be deployed. The best-known option is known as "march-in rights," which can be exercised when "health and safety needs . . . are not being reasonably satisfied" or when the medicine is not "available to the public on reasonable terms."[12] The second option provided by Bayh-Dole is for the federal government to simply exercise its right to use the federally funded invention for its own purposes, without paying royalties to the patent-holder.[13] An obvious use of that second option would be to license the generic manufacture of a drug for use in the Medicare, Medicaid, and other federally supported health programs.[14]

As some medicine-access scholars have put it, "The logic behind using the march-in authority is that taxpayers should not have to pay twice for publicly-funded research—once through taxes, and once through monopoly prices or restricted access to drugs."[15] Bayh-Dole has provided the platform for multiple requests for the National Institutes of Health (NIH) to exercise its right to license the medicines that it helped develop and that were later priced at exorbitant levels or not widely available. Unfortunately, in a testament to the U.S. lobbying power of the pharmaceutical industry, not a single march-in request, or any requests to license a medicine for federal use, has been granted in the thirty-five-plus years since the law was adopted.[16]

The growing public unrest over patented medicine prices in the United States, however, has spurred a new wave of efforts seeking to invoke Bayh-Dole rights. In January of 2016, fifty-one members of the U.S. House of Representatives wrote the NIH and the Department of Health and Human Services (HHS), urging the agencies to consider exercising their legal authority. "When drugs are developed with taxpayer funds, the government can and should act to bring relief from out-of-control drug pricing," said Representative Lloyd Doggett (D-TX), a senior member of the House Ways and Means Committee. "There is a difference between earning a profit and profiteering. The Administration should use every tool it has to rein in the practice of pricing a drug at whatever the sick, suffering, or dying will pay."[17] The fifty-one members of Congress chastised the NIH for never taking advantage of march-in or licensing rights in the past, saying the historic reluctance to use the legal remedies "sent an unfortunate signal that prices for federally funded inventions can be set as high as a sick or dying consumer is willing to pay."[18]

Also in 2016, the advocacy groups Knowledge Ecology International and Union for Affordable Cancer Treatment asked the HHS, NIH, and Department of Defense to exercise march-in or federal-use rights on a prostate cancer drug, enzalutamide, invented at the University of California, Los Angeles (UCLA) with research funded by the NIH and Department of Defense. Despite its U.S. provenance, the price charged by the patent-holder of enzalutamide, a Japanese pharmaceutical corporation that markets the drug as Xtandi, is almost $130,000 per year in the United States, as much as four times higher than in other high-income countries.[19] The NIH declined the march-in request, stating only that the medicine was not in short supply.[20] That response was consistent with NIH Director Dr. Francis Collins's April 2016 Senate testimony that the Bayh-Dole rights to license generic production were limited to instances when the product was not "commercialized" and that high prices were irrelevant in determining the right of the government to intervene.[21] That interpretation was challenged at the hearing by Senator Richard Durbin (D-IL), and rightly so: the NIH self-limitation is simply contrary to the legislative history of the law or any reasonable interpretation of it.[22]

In 2015, Senator Bernie Sanders (Ind.-VT) proposed that the U.S. Veterans Administration exercise its compulsory licensing rights, preserved under a U.S. statute similar to Bayh-Dole, to buy generic versions of the patented hepatitis C medicines whose prices were creating a significant financial strain on the agency.[23] The following year, researchers from Yale Law School and Harvard Medical School cited the same hepatitis C medicine crisis when arguing that the U.S. government has rights that are analogous to eminent domain to allow the production of a patented medicine that is priced at unaffordable levels, even when the medicine did not stem from a federally funded discovery.[24] As these scholars, lawmakers, and advocates point out, current law provides a path that leads away from huge prices on prescription drugs in the United States, if only elected officials had the political will to follow that path. As I discuss in the conclusion, activists are now working hard to push elected officials in that direction.

*   *   *

Beyond TRIPS flexibilities at the international level and Bayh-Dole march-in rights in the United States, access-to-medicine advocates have other paths they can follow to pursue more affordable medicines. One of these routes is to put pressure on national governments by adding drugs to the World Health Organization Essential Medicines List. The list acts as a model formulary of the medicines that are important enough that they should be readily available to all, without the price creating a barrier to access.[25] The Essential Medicines List has been around since 1977, but it truly proved its persuasive potential in the early 2000s, when the addition of antiretroviral drugs to the list helped fuel the movement to reduce the price of those lifesaving medicines.[26]

In 2015, advocates successfully concluded a multiyear campaign to add several cancer, tuberculosis, and hepatitis C medicines to the Essential Medicine List, in the hopes that their inclusion would spur pressure to increase their availability.[27] When these medicines, including sixteen additional cancer drugs, were added to the list, advocates called it a "watershed moment."[28] Director-General Dr. Margaret Chan of the World Health Organization, is among those who thinks that optimism is well justified. "When new effective medicines emerge to safely treat serious and widespread diseases, it is vital to ensure that everyone who needs them can obtain them," Chan said when announcing the addition of the new drugs to the list. "Placing them on the WHO Essential Medicines List is a first step in that direction."[29]

Advocates have also found space under existing law to create some negotiating power over monopoly patent pricing, specifically in the form of coordinated purchasing of medicines in bulk. The U.S. President's Emergency Plan for AIDS Relief (PEPFAR), the Pan-American Health Organization, and the Stop TB Partnership all have obtained lower medicine prices by leveraging the bargaining power that comes with their purchasing enormous amounts of medicines for global distribution.[30] The UN-backed Medicines Patent Pool has persuaded corporate patent-holders to license their medicines for generic manufacturing in low- to middle-income countries that do not present promising patent-price markets for the corporations. Using this approach, the pool has helped distribute 3 billion doses of medicines, predominately for HIV/AIDS but now expanding to include hepatitis C, TB, and cancer treatments.[31] Some experts have suggested the Medicines Patent Pool could one day be expanded to cover all essential medicines.[32]

Even the U.S. government has recognized that current international law provides pathways to affordable medicines. In 2007, proposed trade agreements between the United States and Peru and Panama that were negotiated by the George W. Bush administration faced opposition by congressional members of the Democratic Party. The Democrats felt that the deals did not include adequate protections for labor and environmental concerns, as well as access to medicines. The Bush administration and the congressional Democrats reached a compromise, formally titled the "U.S. Bipartisan Compact on Free Trade Agreements" and widely referred to as the May 10th Agreement.

The May 10th Agreement reaffirmed the rights to issue compulsory licenses for needed medicines. Its aim was also to lessen the impact of TRIPS-Plus provisions such as data exclusivity, patent linkage, and evergreening.[33] The May 10th Agreement broke no new legal ground in medicine access because those provisions were already included in the TRIPS and Doha agreements; nevertheless. it did put the U.S. government on record as respecting the patent bypass rights reserved in TRIPS and Doha. The advocacy value of that declaration has been demonstrated recently by medicine activists and members of Congress predicating their opposition to the Trans-Pacific Partnership Agreement in part on the argument that the terms of the agreement violate the pledges contained in the May 10th Agreement.[34]

Governments can also protect against the overuse of medicine patents by more tightly enforcing the requirements that pharmaceutical corporations must meet before they are granted a patent. TRIPS preserves the flexibility of individual nations to determine for themselves when to grant patent applications, specifically the right to decide when those applications meet the requirements for including what is known as an "inventive step."[35]

We recall from chapter 12 the problem of pharmaceutical corporations evergreening their patents by seeking new patents for trivial changes to existing medicines. Under current law, nations are already allowed to follow the lead of countries such as India, which shuts down evergreening efforts by requiring that new forms, uses, or formulations of existing medicines cannot get a new patent unless they enhance "therapeutic efficacy."[36] Tighter enforcement of patent requirements will lead to less evergreening and more access to low-price medicines.

*   *   *

In addition to lowering the prices of medicine by simply taking advantage of existing law, lower medicine prices can be achieved through limited changes to the current rules while still leaving the overall patent regime in place. Most of the reform proposals in this small changes category have been generated by U.S. advocates and politicians. There are two reasons for this. First, the political power of the pharmaceutical industry in the United States is so imposing that more radical reforms are considered de facto off the table by most elected officials.[37] Second, the uniquely hands-off approach to monopoly medicine pricing in the United States has led to U.S. patients and providers paying the highest medicine prices in the world.[38] As one journalist put it, "We are the only developed nation that lets drug makers set their own prices—maximizing profits the same way that sellers of chairs, mugs, shoes, or any other seller of manufactured goods would."[39]

U.S. costs per capita for medicines are more than twice the average of other high-income countries.[40] The resulting frustration among U.S. voters is so pronounced that the medicine status quo is criticized even by U.S. politicians who ordinarily oppose government regulation. For example, Senator Marco Rubio (R-FL), a 2016 presidential candidate, labeled some drug pricing as "pure profiteering" that could "bankrupt" the U.S. system, and President Donald Trump vowed in that same campaign to take on the pharma lobby.[41] A bipartisan Senate Special Committee held a hearing in late 2015 focused on drug pricing, citing a crisis triggered by the sudden 500+ percent hikes in some heart and kidney medicines.[42] Also in late 2015, the Obama administration held a high-profile forum on drug pricing.[43] At this writing in mid-2016, the Justice Department is reported to be investigating Big Pharma pricing strategies and antitrust issues, and the FDA is increasing its scrutiny of the clinical data submitted by drug makers.[44]

Perhaps the lowest-hanging fruit for meaningful medicine-pricing reform in the United States would be the repeal of a 2003 law that prohibits the Medicare system, which counts 48 million Americans under its coverage, from negotiating the price of the medicines it pays for.[45] For several years, the Obama administration has pushed for congressional approval for Medicare to negotiate these drug purchases, a change that could save U.S. taxpayers $15 billion annually.[46] Of course, the same pharmaceutical corporations that employed their lobbying heft to create the 2003 law, and to defend the non-negotiable price-setting during the debates over the Affordable Care Act, are directing the same energy and influence to oppose any repeal.[47] In a 2016 essay in the *Journal of the American Medical Association*, President Obama criticized the pharmaceutical industry for its opposition to health care reform before and after the Affordable Care Act was passed, noting the importance of tackling the influence of "special interest dollars in politics."[48]

Despite the resistance from the industry, allowing Medicare to negotiate drug purchases is hardly a radical idea. The practice would follow the lead of other high-income nations that enjoy significantly less expensive medicine prices than the United States pays. For example, some cancer treatments cost five times more in the United States than what the identical treatments cost in Canada, where drug prices are negotiated by the government.[49] Not surprisingly, negotiation of drug prices is an idea that has broad support among people in the United States who struggle to afford their prescriptions. A 2016 poll by the Kaiser Family Foundation found that 82 percent of Americans favored allowing the federal government to negotiate with drug makers.[50] Both major candidates for U.S. president in 2016 supported the idea, including the eventual winner, Donald Trump.[51]

Even U.S. health care CEOs, leaders in a health system that is more privatized than any in the world, are overwhelmingly in favor of unshackling the negotiating power of their government; 86 percent of those leaders responded to a 2015 poll with support for federal authority to bargain for Medicare drug prices. "Historically I'm not a big fan of government intervention in business," said one of the CEOs surveyed. "But I think some intervention on the part of government—whether it is on price-setting or price increases—I think could definitely help people out."[52]

The reference to government price-setting reflects the common practice in other high-income countries, where the government adopts price ceilings based on the therapeutic value of the medicines. For example, the Pharmaceutical Management Agency (PHARMAC) in New Zealand keeps medicine prices low by conducting price negotiations with the patent-holding pharmaceutical companies. It also employs therapeutic reference pricing, which sets the price paid for medicines by comparing them with other medicines with similar therapeutic benefits.[53] These ceilings bring a much-needed medical context to pricing, a context that is absent from the whatever-the-market-will-bear monopoly medicine pricing described in chapter 9.[54] Not surprisingly, governments that adopt such ceilings create bargaining power that leads to significantly lower medicine prices. And analysis of the drug development history in those nations shows that the lower prices have been obtained without sacrificing medicine innovation.[55]

Another popular U.S. reform proposal calls for shining a light on to the hidden world of pharmaceutical corporate finances, specifically by requiring transparency from the corporations that reap huge profits from government purchases of their products.[56] As we have seen in chapter 6, there are significant discrepancies between the claims made by the industry about its research and development investment and independent analyses of those costs.[57] Lawmakers at the federal level and in multiple states, including New York, California, Pennsylvania, Texas, North Carolina, Massachusetts, and Oregon, propose requiring manufacturers to reveal their true research and development costs, along with their marketing and advertising expenditures and the profits they make from government-purchased drugs.[58] As a supportive 2015 editorial in the *Los Angeles Times* said, these measures are a long overdue effort to "pry open the healthcare black box."[59] A similar call for medicine cost transparency has been made at the Parliamentary Assembly of the Council of Europe.[60]

There are many other U.S.-focused reform ideas to curb excesses of the medicine patent system, including the following:

• Limiting the U.S. tax deductions allowed for pharmaceutical corporation advertising costs
• Reducing the length of medicine patents
• Allowing patients to personally import cheaper medicines from Canada
• Cracking down on patent evergreening
• Regulating the pharmaceutical industry as a utility, including the creation of price review boards[61]

In addition, the American Medical Association recently convened a task force that called for a shortened exclusivity period for biologics, greater monitoring of pharmaceutical corporation mergers and acquisitions, and increased cost transparency.[62] The American Hospital Association and multiple insurers chimed in with their own calls for greater transparency in drug pricing and research and development costs.[63] All these reforms would have the effect of lowering medicine prices with relatively minor changes to existing law.

21

THERE IS A BETTER WAY
TO DEVELOP MEDICINES

I have discussed in chapter 20 how small but significant changes can be easily accomplished under current law or with small tweaks to it. Here I review how to make more substantial fixes to our broken system.

When pharmaceutical corporations defend the current patent medicine system, they say that the massive profits generated from monopoly pricing are necessary to provide the incentive for the research and development of new medicines. This argument should not be dismissed lightly: on behalf of anyone facing a diagnosis of terminal or incurable illness, and on behalf of their loved ones, the search for new medicines is a life-or-death priority. But, as we have seen in chapter 14, government funding, not private dollars, provides the foundation for that kind of research. And those government funds can provide incentives for drug development without the deadly side effects of patent monopolies.

Most comprehensive medicine-development reform proposals provide those incentives using some combination of "push" and "pull" mechanisms.[1] Push incentives include grants or other subsidies offered to innovators at the early stage of medicine research. Governments are already playing the most critical role in this early-stage medicine research. The most prominent example of push funding is the substantial investment by the NIH, which provides $32 billion annually in government funding for medical research. The long list of NIH success stories includes supporting the work of 148 Nobel Prize winners, along with the funding of the research that led to the antiretroviral medicines that revolutionized the treatment of HIV/AIDS and saved millions of lives worldwide.[2]

Beyond the NIH, an example of smaller but more targeted push funding is the Drugs for Neglected Diseases Initiative, a not-for-profit collaboration among the public sector, academia, nongovernmental organizations, and for-profit companies.[3] Under the Drugs for Neglected Diseases Initiative umbrella, this coalition spurs research and development for neglected diseases. It now has more than thirty projects in its research and development pipeline, including fifteen entirely new chemical entities.[4] The success of the Drugs for Neglected Diseases Initiative, as well as that of the Italian Mario Negri Institute, which refuses to take patents on its discoveries, has helped spur calls in Europe for an expansion in nonprofit medicine research and development.[5] Also in the push category are government-provided tax credits for pharmaceutical research, credits that are sometimes increased to reward research that addresses diseases with limited profit potential.[6]

When governments provide push funding, they can and should be requiring that the resulting knowledge be made public and available to all in an open access database.[7] That approach will reverse the anti-innovation character of patents and tear down the many isolated secretive silos of current patent medicine research. It is exciting to contemplate the prospects for global health when the proven power of open sourcing is unleashed to tackle the most vexing health challenges of our time.

In contrast, pull funding usually focuses on the later stages of the research and development process. The most widely discussed pull proposals center on offering significant prizes to innovators who discover and develop a valuable drug.[8] Such prizes are certainly not a new idea; there is a long history of prizes being used to spur innovation. Architectural design prizes, for example, date back to the fifteenth century. And Charles Lindbergh's famous 1927 trans-Atlantic flight earned him the $25,000 Orteig prize.[9]

In fact, the current medicine patent system is itself a prize model. The problem is that the prize of a monopoly market leads to bloated prices and siloed research, and it fails to provide incentives for the development of medicines that address diseases that plague the global poor. Therefore, most modern medicine-development prize proposals include, as a condition of acceptance, an open-source commitment: the release of any monopoly rights to the medicine formula.[10]

Just as with conditional push funding, the expectation is that the resulting open development of prize-induced medicines will lead to low-cost manufacturing and innovations in delivery methods. This is much more than wishful thinking because that kind of innovation already characterizes the current generic drug industry, in which formulas are not locked away from those who wish to improve on them.[11]

The Health Impact Fund is one prize proposal that has attracted high-profile supporters, including Amatrya Sen, Nobel laureate economist; Dr. Paul Farmer, global health activist; and Peter Singer, philosopher. The plan of the fund is to offer drug developers prizes in amounts that correspond to the impact of their innovation on global health. In return for the prizes, recipients surrender any rights to monopoly pricing, which means that drug prices will be more closely linked to the costs of manufacture.[12]

The Health Impact Fund and most other medicine prize proposals are still on the drawing board, but some prize programs are already in place. Those include a European Union prize for vaccines innovation, the National Health Service England Innovation Challenge Prizes, and the Longitude Prize for developing antibiotics.[13] As health economists have noted, the structure of these prize programs does not present a radical change to the current medicines research model. As we have seen in chapter 6, much of the current private-sector innovation comes from small research firms, whose "prize" is having their most successful projects bought up by large pharmaceutical corporations.[14] There are examples of medicine development prizes that are funded by private philanthropy in whole or in part, but substantial government investment will be necessary for prizes to replace the lucrative rewards of a patent monopoly.

The same is true for related pull proposals, such as advanced purchase commitments that provide incentives for drug development by guaranteeing a market for a medicine that may not otherwise appear profitable to an innovator.[15] As with push funding, the need for substantial government investment in pull programs does not pose as much of a challenge as it may initially appear: the government dollars needed for prize systems or advanced purchase commitments already undergird the current patent system. Governments pay at both the push and pull stages already in the form of the public funding of research followed by high-volume government purchases of patent-priced medicines.[16] In the United States, for example, Medicare and Medicaid programs now purchase many drugs at patent prices, including the drugs the government paid to develop.

We simply need to change the direction of those government funds to benefit patients rather than enrich corporations. If we just commit to that switch in priorities, there is more than enough money in the current system to finance medicine research and development.[17] As an added bonus, that government investment would not be handcuffed by for-profit priorities that neglect major diseases in favor of maladies that impact the comparatively wealthy. Further savings would be realized by the elimination of the need for medicine prices to be set high enough to recoup the cost of for-profit drug marketing. The five largest US pharmaceutical companies spend a combined $50 billion annually on marketing, an expense that currently gets passed on to medicine purchasers.[18] We can do without that!

When considering how to provide incentives for medicine research, it is important to realize that different stages of medicine research and development pose different challenges. Effective incentives to spur basic research may not work to motivate the launch of clinical trials, which are currently conducted largely by private corporations but are often beset with profit-connected ethical problems.[19] As a result, many reformers advocate the use of a combination of push and pull approaches. For example, Médicins Sans Frontières/Doctors Without Borders is pursuing a 3P project—push, pull, and pooling (sharing of research results)—to develop an effective TB treatment.[20]

Another well-known example of combining push and pull incentives is the U.S. Orphan Drug Act. This law was introduced to spur research to find medicines to address diseases whose remedies are not likely to produce a huge profit for the manufacturer, usually because the diseases affect a small number of people. The Orphan Drug Act provides an early-stage push, in the form of research grants and increased tax credits, along with a late-stage pull from government-guaranteed market exclusivity for the resulting drugs.[21] Australia and the European Union have created similar push-pull mechanisms to stimulate the research and development of medicines that target rare (orphan) diseases.[22]

James Love, the director of the medicine-access group Knowledge Ecology International, is a former longshoreman turned community activist who then decided to study economics, eventually becoming a staffer for Ralph Nader, the famed consumer advocate.[23] Love played a key role in convincing Indian generic drug manufacturer Cipla to make a dramatic 2001 pledge to manufacture and sell antiretroviral medicines at a cost of $1 per day.[24] That offer of a 96 percent reduction from the patented price gained immediate international attention, put pressure on both drug companies and governments to respond to the HIV/AIDS pandemic, and helped lead to a huge expansion in HIV/AIDS treatment.

Love and his organization are known for in-depth analyses of proposed drug regulations and the profits and research investments of the pharmaceutical industry. He was instrumental in devising the UN-backed Medicines Patent Pool (chapter 20), in which companies have voluntarily surrendered their monopolies on antiretrovirals in poor countries in return for royalties on cheaply produced generic versions.

The Medicines Patent Pool has been a success. But Love and other medicine advocates point out that there is a ceiling on such a plan. After all, pharmaceutical companies will voluntarily surrender their patents only in countries where they know they cannot sell their drugs at higher costs. "The pool is a transition thing," Love said. "The transformative change comes with delinkage."[25]

Delinkage is the term used to describe a set of proposals that breaks the connection between medicine prices and the costs of research and development. Many of the reform proposals we have mentioned include meaningful alterations to the current medicines patent model. But most do not completely delink medicine prices from research costs, nor do they discard the existing patent system. The Medicines Patent Pool, for example, does not disturb the rights of the patent-holders to charge monopoly prices in middle- and high-income countries. Similarly, the aim of the Health Impact Fund is the patent-free development and distribution of drugs for neglected diseases only. It does not affect the ability of the patent-holders to charge monopoly prices for medicines with high market values, which includes many cancer medicines.

In contrast, Love and others call for the complete delinkage of medicine prices from the costs of research and development. The aim of delinkage proposals is to support research for needed medicines while bypassing the need for patients to pay for the enormous marketing costs now poured into noncritical drugs and "me-too" variations of existing medicines. "The amount of marketing goes up with the unimportance of the drug," Love says. "You don't have to convince people of the value of antiretrovirals or a cancer drug that saves lives."[26]

An example of a full delinkage proposal is the Medical Innovation Prize Fund proposed by Love and others, which would reward innovations that impact public health while requiring the surrender of all monopoly patent rights.[27] Under proposals such as these, medicine prices would closely correspond to manufacturing costs, which are often quite inexpensive. The idea of delinkage is grounded in both the pre-TRIPS history of treating medicines as a public good (chapter 16) and the modern acknowledgement of the human right to health (chapter 22).

Under delinkage, one aspect of the current drug research model would remain intact. Love insists that any medicine development program has to include sufficient monetary incentives to entice research from the private sector. Love's wife, Manon Ress, also an intellectual property expert and activist, has Stage IV breast cancer. Love points out that patients like her—and loved ones like him—understandably want the search for new medicines to be aggressive and relentless. And if that research is done by the pharmaceutical companies that currently embrace the patent model, so much the better. "If you do the delinkage right, with real rewards for innovation, the companies that are good at innovation will do just fine," Love says.[28] Others agree. Writing in the prestigious British medical journal *The Lancet,* World Health Organization leaders discussed how the private sector could play the role of government contractors in a publicly-funded medicines system.[29] Economist Dean Baker has promoted this model, comparing it to the existing system of government defense contracting to private companies to conduct research and develop products, an arrangement that Baker points out has led to ground-breaking technological advances.[30]

The escalating global outrage over the flaws in the current medicine monopoly system is allowing these delinkage arguments to gain traction.[31] An August 2015 article in the *Economist* conducted a thorough and skeptical review of the value of patents for medicines, concluding that reform proposals deserve an opportunity to demonstrate whether they can provide better results than the current system.[32] The concept of delinkage received an extensive and favorable review in a 2013 joint report of the WTO, the World Intellectual Property Organization, and the World Health Organization, and in a 2016 report from an expert international panel convened by the British medical journal *The Lancet.*[33] "I'm absolutely optimistic that there can be big changes, and soon," Love says. "We just need to get the messaging right, and we need the political leadership to step up. I mean, the benefits are so obvious."[34]

An important opportunity for the global political leadership to heed Love's call to step up was presented by the convening of the UN Secretary-General's High-Level Panel on Access to Medicines, announced in late 2015. Human rights advocates, however, have learned to approach with restraint the news of a high-profile group convening to review a crisis: too often, such groups issue a promising report that is ignored or, worse, completely contradicted by binding trade agreements that elevate corporate profits over human rights.[35]

But human rights history also gives us reason for some optimism. That history shows that discussions about a right usually goes on for decades, if not generations, before it becomes an enforceable reality. Plenty of blue-ribbon panels were convened and reports written along the path to overcoming slavery, apartheid, and colonialism—even though it took more pro-active in-the-street and in-your-face protests, boycotts, and political action to put those movements over the top.

As for this particular panel, its membership was undeniably impressive. Notably, it included Yusuf Hamied, the chair of the generic drug manufacturer Cipla who worked with James Love and others to make sure that low-cost generic medicines helped fuel the historically successful HIV/AIDS treatment movement.[36] There were politicians and a Big Pharma CEO on the panel, too, but other members include Winnie Byanyima of Oxfam and Stephen Lewis, a veteran Canadian diplomat and HIV/AIDS treatment activist. Lewis has seen such panels come and go without having much impact, but he believed that this time might be different. "Access to medicines has become one of humankind's greatest crises, perhaps right behind climate change," he said in December 2015. "This has become a problem for the developed world alongside the developing world, and I think that means great changes are coming."[37]

Lewis's fellow panel members seemed to recognize the problem as well. The panel ultimately issued a report that began with a clear recognition that millions die each year from AIDS, TB, hepatitis C, and noncommunicable diseases, all due to lack of access to medicines that would have saved their lives.[38] The report also affirmed the fundamental right to access medicines and vaccines, and that there is abundant evidence to show that the market alone cannot be trusted to provide lifesaving medicines.[39]

Ultimately, the panel issued a strong call for governments to exercise their existing legal rights to pursue generic manufacturing of unaffordable patented medicines and tightly restrict medicine patents and extensions. Two-thirds of the panel supported a process to allow immediate generic manufacture of all essential medicines, although consensus was not reached on that point.[40] But the whole panel did not shy away from making the big-picture recommendation that the secretary-general and UN member states should work toward a binding research and development convention (agreement). That convention would delink the price of medicines from the cost of research and development, a necessary step toward treating essential medicines as a core component of the human right to health instead of a for-profit commodity ripe for exploitation.[41]

The suggestion for an international agreement on medicines research and price is not a new one. In 2012, a working group created by the World Health Assembly, the decision-making body of the World Health Organization, issued a report proposing a binding treaty to enforce government funding of health-related research and development. The proposal called for all countries to spend at least 0.01 percent of their gross domestic product on neglected diseases.[42]

Under the proposed treaty terms, 20 percent of this investment would be pooled at the international level, but some could be directed by individual nations toward early-stage research, prize funds, patent buy-outs, or other push-pull mechanisms. The treaty was designed to lay the platform for open-source development of the next generation of medicines. But the United States led opposition to the treaty during the 2012 World Health Organization discussions, and the consideration of the proposal was postponed.[43]

After that postponement, a renewed effort to push a global research and development pact was organized by Universities Allied for Essential

Medicines (UAEM), a student-led global organization that has traditionally focused on promoting wide access to university-developed medicines.[44] Beginning in 2015, the students decided to set their sights more broadly. "On the whole, patent monopolies have proven to be the wrong incentive for research and development of medical products to meet global health needs," the students said in a UAEM report. "Delinking the price of drugs from their R&D costs (is necessary) in order to delink the main incentive for their production from a market base and bring it back to public interest."[45]

The foundation for the current global push for a research and development agreement has been a November 2015 letter to the World Health Organization signed by dozens of academics and scientists, including two Nobel laureates. "Patent monopolies increasingly enable rising drug prices, without any corresponding increase in innovation," they wrote the World Health Organization. "We have witnessed stagnation in the face of public health emergencies."[46] The letter favorably cited current prize funds, patent pools, and open-source efforts, but it also noted that these efforts are fragmented. "A global agreement for an equitable biomedical R&D system can provide a much needed structure," the signers wrote. "It can provide guiding principles which can move us to a system that incentivizes research and technology transfer based on global health needs and recognizes the human right to health."[47] Many others have endorsed the idea of a global research and development agreement, including the essential medicines panel convened in 2016 by *The Lancet*, which noted precedent for such an agreement provided by the impactful 2005 Framework Convention on Tobacco Control.[48] The members of the World Health Organization did not adopt the global agreement during their 2016 meeting, but they did agree on a resolution calling for more examination of a pooled research and development funding model, leading advocates to be hopeful that a global research funding agreement would still be possible.[49]

Admittedly, delinkage proposals, including the global research and development agreement, are not without complexities and challenges. Push funding requires rigorous compliance monitoring and cannot guarantee success for every effort to discover innovative medicines. For prize systems, it is not easy to determine a monetary value and terms that will provide sufficient motivation for innovators, along with robust returns for the prize funders.

But none of the possible limitations of reform proposals approaches the fatal dysfunction of the present skewed reward system, which causes needless suffering and death. The medicine patent system produces toxic results, and medicine advocates have come together to support effective and equitable alternatives. These alternatives deserve global support.

22

HUMAN RIGHTS LAW DEMANDS ACCESS TO ESSENTIAL MEDICINES

As part of my law school faculty duties, I teach classes in human rights law. If I wanted to do so—and if my students would put up with it—we could spend several weeks of class just describing the many sources of law that establish a human right to health, including the right to essential medicines.

We would start by recognizing that the idea that individuals possess human rights is one that existed long before there were international treaties and institutions designed to define and protect those rights.[1] Those international treaties are relatively new, with most dating back only to the mid-twentieth century. But there is a long history of human rights, including the human right to health, being well respected stretching back for generations before these formal treaties ever existed.

All major religious traditions, and virtually all philosophical approaches, which have long had an enormous impact on the law, set out a clear mandate to provide for the needs of the poor and sick. Most have done so using language that invokes justice and rights, not merely charity. Old

Testament prophets and Jesus Christ spoke in terms of justice, often in the context of addressing the needs of the sick.[2] The Qur'an speaks passionately of justice, and Confucian principles embrace a community-wide obligation to provide for the needs of all.[3] St. Augustine said that charity cannot make up for justice withheld.[4]

Following in those religious and moral traditions, many individual governments in Europe and the United States have long embraced a responsibility to provide for health care and what are known as the "social determinants of health," which include universal subsistence needs such as food and water and shelter.[5] In the early twentieth century, the constitutions of Mexico, the Soviet Union, and the Weimar Republic all articulated a governmental obligation to address economic and social needs.[6] On the international level, the Treaty of Versailles in 1919 created the International Labour Organization, which eventually adopted standards that included insurance in the event of injury, illness, and old age.[7]

In the United States, some state constitutions adopted in the nineteenth and twentieth centuries articulated rights to health and general welfare.[8] Beginning in the nineteenth century, states implemented government poor relief programs.[9] And in the 1930s, New Deal legislation created ambitious and successful federal programs designed to address the social determinants of health, including social security to meet the needs of the sick and disabled.[10]

In President Franklin Roosevelt's 1944 State of the Union address, he sought to build on the success of that New Deal legislation and the impending end of World War II by laying out an agenda he called a Second Bill of Rights. Prominent among those rights was "The right to adequate medical care and the opportunity to achieve and enjoy good health."[11] Roosevelt's Second Bill of Rights followed his 1941 State of the Union address outlining the Four Freedoms: freedom of speech, freedom of worship, freedom from want, and freedom from fear.[12]

These Roosevelt speeches animated the deliberations of the new United Nations when it created the Constitution of the World Health Organization in 1946 and the Universal Declaration of Human Rights in 1948. Both these documents made clear that all individuals in the world possess the fundamental right to the highest attainable standard of health.[13] The qualifier *highest attainable standard* reflects the fact that it is impossible for a government to guarantee good health. Although health is largely determined by social determinants such as food, water, and safety, along with access to care and medicines in a time of need, some health issues, attributable to genetics or personal choice, are outside the control of a government.

But access to medicines is most definitely something a government can influence. So, in 1978, the world's nations adopted the Declaration of Alma-Ata on Primary Health Care, which listed essential drugs as one of the components of primary health care, identified by the representatives of 134 nations as "a most important world-wide social goal."[14] The International Covenant on Economic, Social and Cultural Rights (ICESCR) builds on the nonbinding Universal Declaration of Human Rights by imposing in its Article 12 the obligation for state parties to take steps to achieve the full realization of the right to health.[15]

The UN Committee on Economic, Social and Cultural Rights (ESCR Committee) has the task of explaining in more detail what governments are obligated to do to fulfill this right. Chiefly through the 2000 document General Comment No. 14, the committee made it clear that one core and immediate obligation is ensuring the availability, accessibility, and good quality of essential medicines.[16] The ICESCR is an all-but-universal treaty, with 164 countries having signed on. Unfortunately, the United States is one of just a handful of countries that has not yet ratified the ICESCR. But the United States is a party to the Universal Declaration of Human Rights, the Constitution of the World Health Organization, and other international agreements and declarations that establish a clear right to health.[17]

Whenever that right to health is described by major human rights organizations, access to essential medicines is front and center. The UN high commissioner for human rights includes access to essential medicines as one of five indicators of the fulfillment by a country of the right to health and has urged states to pursue policies that facilitate the purchase of low-cost generic medicines.[18] The World Health Organization has created a Department of Essential Medicines and Pharmaceutical Policies, and it has firmly stated that the right to access essential medicines is well-founded in international law.[19] The Human Rights Council, which is composed of UN member countries elected by the UN General Assembly, has confirmed that the right to health includes access to medicines and that such rights supersede interests in international trade, investment, and intellectual property.[20] That position was unequivocally repeated in 2016 by the UN High-Level Panel on Access to Medicines, which stated in its final report, "Human rights are fundamental, universal entitlements that people inherently acquire by virtue of their birth. In comparison, intellectual property rights . . . are temporary, revocable, transferrable privileges granted by states and can be suspended or revoked."[21]

At a national level, most countries have explicitly recognized the human right to the highest attainable standard of health within their own borders, whether by signing international and regional treaties or by laying out the right to health in their national constitutions—or, in many cases, both.[22] These are not just empty promises. Many courts across the globe have issued rulings recognizing the right to health, including the right to access to medicine, and ordering that the right be fulfilled by governments.[23]

We know from chapter 18 that trade agreements usually work to protect medicine monopolies and against access to affordable medicines. So, it is important to realize that, as a matter of human rights law, those trade deals do not stand on equal footing with the human rights obligations of any country. Although the Universal Declaration and the ICESCR include the right to protection of an inventor's "moral and material interests" in a scientific, literary, or artistic product, the ICESCR also guarantees a human right to "enjoy the benefits of a scientific program and its applications."[24]

In 2006, the ESCR Committee cleared up any potential conflict between intellectual property rights and human rights, stating that it is important not to equate the two. Expressly citing the human right to essential medicine and specifically calling out the patent regime, the committee said, "States parties should prevent the use of scientific and technical progress for purposes contrary to human rights and dignity, including the rights to life, health and privacy, e.g. by excluding inventions from patentability whenever their commercialization would jeopardize the full realization of these rights."[25]

This do-no-harm requirement for countries includes the duty to actively prevent third parties—such as pharmaceutical companies—from taking actions that would have a negative effect on human rights, such as access to medicines. This commitment is binding on governments even when that harm would be felt in other countries, which is clearly the case whenever the United States pushes trade agreement terms that increase patent rights and reduce access to medicine.[26] The bottom line is this: in the eyes of the law, when the human right to health clashes with intellectual property rights, the human right to health wins.

Of course, it is no secret that TRIPS-Plus trade agreements (chapter 18) set the stage for violations of the human right to essential medicine. That problem was specifically addressed by the ESCR Committee in 1999, when it reminded the World Trade Organization that trade liberalization should serve the goals of international human rights instruments.[27] In 2009, the UN special rapporteur on the right to health strongly criticized the TRIPS-Plus agreements for undermining the right to access essential medicines.[28]

More recently, a group of UN experts issued a 2015 statement that addressed access to medicines and TPP and TTIP. "Observers are concerned that these treaties and agreements are likely to have a number of retrogressive effects on the protection and promotion of human rights, including . . . by catering to the business interests of pharmaceutical monopolies and extending intellectual property protection."[29]

Although human rights documents chiefly impose obligations on governments, pharmaceutical corporations have human rights responsibilities as well. The ESCR Committee 2000 General Comment No. 14 lays out corporate obligations, as do the UN Guiding Principles on Business and Human Rights. Both explicitly admonish businesses to avoid actions that would cause adverse human rights impacts.[30]

Yet, as we know, the pharmaceutical corporations have ignored these mandates. The UN special rapporteur on the right to the highest attainable standard of health also knows that, so in 2008 he issued a very specific report on this issue, entitled "Human Rights Guidelines for Pharmaceutical Companies in Relation to Access to Medicines."[31] Stating that enhancing access to medicines has "the central place in the societal mission of pharmaceutical companies," and noting the benefits the industry receives from government-paid research and government-provided patent protections, the special rapporteur outlined recommendations that corporations contribute to the research and development for neglected diseases, and refrain from efforts to block access to essential medicines.

The special rapporteur's guidelines include cooperating with countries that seek to provide their populations with the benefits of patented medicines through compulsory licensing and importation of affordable generic medicines. The special rapporteur also discouraged pharmaceutical corporations from lobbying for increased protection of their intellectual property interests when that protection would negatively affect access to essential medicines. The special rapporteur recognized that this negative impact occurs as a result of patent-elongating schemes such as data exclusivity and evergreening.[32]

In sum, the human right to health, including the human right to essential medicines, is unequivocal and well established. Yet this human right has proven to be very difficult to enforce. Well-funded powerful corporations and governments have put up roadblock after roadblock on the path to universal access to affordable medicines.

But that this human right to essential medicines is not yet being well enforced does not change the fact that it exists, anymore than the continued existence of slavery in the world calls into question the human right to freedom. In the conclusion of this book I focus on how the human right to essential medicines can be made a reality in the lives of all people.

CONCLUSION

We have made the mightiest industry in the world shake in its boots!
—ZACKIE ACHMAT, TREATMENT ACTION CAMPAIGN

The turn of the twenty-first century featured some very positive news in HIV/AIDS treatment.[1] Recently discovered antiretroviral medicines (ARVs) had been proven to be hugely effective in combatting the virus. In fact, ARVs were so potent that their impact on patients was known as the Lazarus effect: people with AIDS were literally rising from what all had presumed would be their deathbeds.[2] Suddenly, HIV/AIDS was transformed from a death sentence into a chronic but manageable disease—for those who could afford the medicine.[3]

But that miracle medicine was protected by patents held by multinational pharmaceutical companies, despite the fact that government-supported scientists played the key roles in discovering the drugs and developing their potential for use in HIV/AIDS therapy.[4] The price of the ARVs established by the companies was over $1,000 per month, prohibitively expensive for patients and governments in low-income countries.[5] As is typically the case with patent-protected medicines, that price tag bore no resemblance to the production cost of the medicines, which was barely over $1 per daily dose.[6]

By 2000, ARV treatment had become widely available across North American and Europe, but just 1 of every 1,000 Africans infected with HIV had access to the medicines.[7] The impact of this lack of treatment was staggering: more than 2 million Africans were dying from AIDS each year.[8]

South Africa was particularly hard hit, with the prevalence of HIV as high as 25 percent among women of childbearing age.[9] In 2000, more South Africans died in their thirties and forties than did in their sixties and seventies.[10] In neighboring Zimbabwe, morgues began staying open twenty-four hours a day to receive the bodies that were being brought in at all hours.[11] Yet, largely due to the monopoly pricing of the medicines, the conventional wisdom was that it was not going to be possible to treat HIV in the developing world. "It's so politically incorrect to say, but we may have to sit by and just see these millions of people die," an unnamed global health official told the *Washington Post* in early 2001.[12]

I am sad to say that I had my own experience doing just that. Shortly after the turn of the century, I visited Moi Teaching and Referral Hospital in Eldoret, Kenya. Although some HIV/AIDS medicine was then being provided to a few individuals in the area, the medicine was limited to those whose disease had not advanced. That meant that the women I met at the hospital were going to die without ARV treatment.[13]

One woman, Theresa,[14] lay huddled under a thin blanket in a bed on Ward One of the hospital, a bed she shared with another woman whose feet lay by Theresa's head. She looked up vacantly at the doctors and medical students surrounding her. Theresa was so thin—*wasted* was the term the Kenyan medical student used when reading aloud from his examination notes—that her eyes seemed to bulge out from above her sunken cheeks. The medical student read on. Theresa had had a persistent cough for four years. Her breathing was rapid but shallow. Her mouth and throat were choked with a white fungus that made it appear Theresa had been chewing cotton—it was oral thrush, an indicator of late-stage HIV. Theresa's breathing was so labored because she also had pneumocystis carinii pneumonia, one of the most common and serious infections for people with HIV. The medical student closed by reciting the social history.

Theresa was a twenty-eight-year-old widow with three children at home, the youngest just three years old.

Theresa had plenty of company on the ward. Women lay two or even three to a bed, flies alighting on their heads. We stepped around a woman curled up on the bare floor, clutching herself and moaning. We saw Elizabeth, who had arms the circumference of a broom handle. Janet was in a coma, Beatrice had skin lesions.

Alice had not been tested yet, but she showed signs of late-stage HIV and had lost her husband to the disease a few years before. As we stood by her bedside, I was bumped in my hip. I turned to see an attendant trying to maneuver a rickety aluminum cart past me. On the cart was a small body under a stained blanket. For all these patients, that would be their fate soon enough. It was a horrifying scene, and one being reproduced thousands of times a day across the African continent.

Against this grim backdrop, a small South African group calling itself the Treatment Action Campaign (TAC) was formed. Its first effort, on Human Rights Day in 1998, consisted of ten people fasting in front of St. George's Cathedral in Cape Town, asking passersby to sign a petition demanding the government provide medicine for pregnant women with HIV/AIDS.[15] But even though TAC had humble beginnings, it possessed excellent organizational genes. Several of its founding members had been active in the anti-apartheid movement, and the group had received training from ACT-UP and other veterans of the passionate, dramatic U.S.-based AIDS treatment campaign of the 1980s and 1990s.[16]

One of the lessons TAC learned from the U.S. activists was the strategy of treatment literacy, in which HIV-vulnerable people in South Africa trained their colleagues in the science and politics of HIV.[17] That training empowered previously marginalized South Africans to mobilize in ambitious campaigns built around direct action, political pressure, and litigation.[18] As TAC co-founder Mark Heywood described it, "People with AIDS ceased being silent victims and became political agitators for their human rights to treatment."[19] The role of the patient-activist moved the medicines issue from an abstract discussion of intellectual property laws to a human rights question. As one HIV-positive TAC activist said at a filmed protest event, "You are denying me drugs. Look me in the face and tell me to die."[20]

TAC soon launched a campaign of civil disobedience, illegally but openly importing a generic version of the AIDS medicine fluconazole. Activists brought the drugs from Thailand, where generic versions cost less than 10 percent of the price charged in South Africa by the patent-holder Pfizer.[21] TAC also proved to be effective at combining legal challenges with the power of mass mobilization.[22] When lawyers argued against the high prices charged for patented medicines or pushed for ramped-up government programming, the courtrooms were packed and the streets outside were filled with thousands of singing, chanting demonstrators.[23] Activists also conducted "die-ins," and even filed charges of culpable homicide against the minister of health.[24]

The face of TAC was its co-founder, Zackie Achmat, who was HIV-positive but refused to take ARVs until they were widely available to the poor of the country. As a result, Achmat suffered through life-threatening lung infections, but he stuck to his vow even after South African President Nelson Mandela personally begged him to take the medicines.[25] Achmat and other TAC activists wore t-shirts with the words "HIV-Positive" in large block letters on the front. The shirts were created after Gugu Dlamini, an AIDS activist, was beaten and stoned to death after revealing her disease status on a radio show. Based loosely on the apocryphal story of the king of Denmark wearing a yellow star in solidarity with Jews during the Nazi occupation, the "HIV-Positive" shirt was worn by individuals irrespective of their status.[26] In December 2002, Mandela wore the shirt during a visit to an AIDS clinic.[27]

When the International AIDS Conference was held in Durban in July 2000, TAC led over 6,000 protestors in a march to the site of the opening ceremonies. The conference hall pulsated with the sound of drums and singing, and a small HIV-positive boy named Nkosi Johnson gave a moving talk. He died the next year at age twelve, without having received ARV treatment.[28]

At those same ceremonies, Edwin Cameron, an HIV-positive South African High Court justice, also spoke to the crowd, laying out the moral imperative. "Those of us who live affluent lives, well attended by medical care and treatment, should not ask how Germans or white South Africans could tolerate living in proximity to moral evil. We do so ourselves today, in proximity to the impending illness and death of many millions of people with AIDS," Cameron said. "Available treatments are denied to those who need them for the sake of aggregating corporate wealth for shareholders who by African standards are unimaginably affluent."[29]

These demonstrations and speeches were widely covered in national and international media. Feeling the pressure building, the pharmaceutical companies decided to go on the offensive. Thirty-nine multinational drug companies filed suit to stop the implementation of the South African Medicines and Related Substances Control Amendment Act, a law that opened the door for international importation of generic medicines.[30] Simultaneously with the pharmaceutical lawsuit, the U.S. trade representative accused the South African government of violating international intellectual property laws, placing the country on a watch list that suspended some trade advantages.[31] The United States also filed a formal complaint against the government of Brazil. Citing the Brazilian constitutional right to health, activists there had successfully pushed for a government program that domestically manufactured generic AIDS medicines.[32]

All the while, the pharmaceutical corporations continued to dismiss the possibility of scaling up HIV/AIDS treatment in the developing world. "Trying to put that much money into the system is like pushing on a string," the Pfizer CEO said in 2001. "We couldn't spend that much money if we had it."[33] As part of its public relations response, pharmaceutical corporations also claimed that generic medicines were of poor quality and that ARVs would not work for Africans.[34]

TAC and global AIDS treatment activists kept up their efforts. Al Gore, U.S. vice president and 2000 presidential candidate, had been an enthusiastic supporter of the tactics of the pharmaceutical industry in resisting access to generic ARVs. So, employing the classic "name and shame" tactic of human rights advocacy, activists relentlessly heckled Gore at his public appearances. They even interrupted his official presidential campaign announcement, chanting "Gore's Greed Kills" and passing out fliers saying "Vice President Gore Doing Drug Company Dirty Work."[35]

Other demonstrations targeted U.S. Trade Representative Charlene Barshefksy, who was leading the push for sanctions against South Africa and Brazil.[36] The international media began following the story, bringing unwanted attention to the Clinton-Gore administration. Finally, reportedly at the urging of Vice President Gore, President Clinton issued a May 2000 Executive Order pledging that the U.S. trade representative would not interfere with the efforts by African nations to obtain cheaper AIDS medicines.[37]

Nevertheless, the lawsuit by the pharmaceutical companies continued, so the activists now focused their attention on the corporations. On March 5, 2001, the day that oral arguments began on the South African lawsuit, TAC led a Global Day of Action against the corporations. Marchers in major cities carried signs saying, "Stop Medical Apartheid." Others convened mock court hearings in front of the offices of GlaxoSmithKline and Bristol Myers Squibb, finding the companies guilty of murder by blocking affordable drugs. The activists said the corporations had blood on their hands and relabeled them "GlobalSerialKillers" and "Big Murder Syndicate."[38]

Finally, drug company executives admitted that the activist campaign was causing "a public relations disaster" for the industry.[39] Six weeks after the Global Day of Action, the companies dropped their lawsuit, even agreeing to pay the legal fees of the South African government.[40] The United States soon withdrew all its punitive measures against South Africa and Brazil.[41]

In November 2001, in the time-honored tradition of the letter of the law following dutifully behind the demands of effective grassroots activism, governments at the WTO Ministerial Conference adopted the Doha Declaration on TRIPS and Public Health. The Doha Declaration affirmed that the TRIPS agreement must be interpreted "in a manner supportive of WTO members' right to protect public health and, in particular, to promote access to medicines for all."[42] The Doha Declaration sent a powerful message, one heard by fifty-plus developing countries that have since taken advantage of TRIPS flexibilities to bypass the patent system to procure lower-cost generic AIDS medicines for their populations.[43] As one activist put it, the signs once carried by, access-to-medicine protesters had been transcribed right into the text of the Doha Declaration.[44]

Continued legal challenges and protests by TAC led the drug companies to allow generic manufacturing of their patented AIDS drugs in South Africa and allowed the government to create a broad HIV/AIDS treatment plan.[45] Demonstrations continued across the world, including body bags being delivered to the White House in Washington, DC, on World AIDS

Day while celebrities and evangelical Christians lobbied President George W. Bush to expand treatment.[46]

With the introduction of generics, the ARV prices in Africa fell by as much as 99 percent. In 2002, the United Nations created the Global Fund to Fight AIDS, Tuberculosis and Malaria, and in 2003, Bush announced the President's Emergency Plan for AIDS Relief (PEPFAR).[47]

The HIV/AIDS treatment picture had changed quickly and dramatically. In 1999, just 20,000 South Africans were on ARVs; today, nearly 3 million are.[48] Globally, PEPFAR and the Global Fund provide ARV treatment for nearly 16 million people.[49]

After the pharmaceutical industry dropped its South African lawsuit, Zachie Achmat, the TAC leader, told a cheering crowd outside the courtroom, "We have made the mightiest industry in the world shake in its boots!"[50] He was right. Evaluated by the scope of the challenge it faced, the powerful resistance it encountered, and the impact it had on millions of lives, the campaign for access to HIV/AIDS medicines was not just the most successful health rights campaign in history—it is one of the most successful human rights campaigns of any kind. And it provides a model for modern-day advocacy for access to essential medicines.

Pushing for change will not be easy. As the HIV/AIDS treatment activists learned, efforts to enforce the human right to essential medicines face the determined resistance of one of the most powerful and profitable industries in the world. We have already seen (chapter 7) that the pharmaceutical industry devotes a significant chunk of its blockbuster revenues to political lobbying, campaign contributions, and marketing of its overall image, all toward the goal of creating the system that provides its corporations with monopoly profits on necessary medicines.

We have seen that those corporate lobbying efforts paid off in the lead-up to the TRIPS Agreement, as the industry-supporting U.S. government used sticks-and-carrots advocacy to pressure nations that were concerned about access to medicines.[51] The same leverage was employed after TRIPS was signed, pushing many countries to adopt patent-protecting medicine laws even earlier than TRIPS forced them to do so.[52] Now that the global patent regime is in place, this same approach is the template for the efforts by the pharmaceutical industry to preserve it.

A recurring target for those pro-monopoly patent efforts is India, home to the generic drug industry that makes the country the "pharmacy of the developing world." The U.S. government and pharmaceutical manufacturers have filed lawsuits and pulled the levers of global trade to undermine India's access-to-medicine measures.[53] Over two hundred members of the U.S. Congress have written to express opposition to generic drug manufacturing in India, and the pharmaceutical industry and other U.S. business groups created a pro-patent coalition, the Alliance for Fair Trade with India.[54] In 2016, criticizing what it called the weak protection of patent rights by India, PhRMA asked the United States to keep India on a priority watch list that could pave the way for trade sanctions. In its request, PhRMA openly admitted to concerns that India's reluctance to facilitate patent monopolies on essential medicines could serve as a model for other nations.[55]

The U.S. trade representative assented to the PhRMA request, keeping India on the watch list; recall (chapter 17) that this designation indicates the country in question has "serious intellectual property rights deficiencies" that require trade scrutiny.[56] The ratcheting up of pressure on India had its desired effect: soon after the watch list decision, the Indian patent office reversed a decision that had denied the U.S. drug manufacturer Gilead a patent in its hepatitis C medicine, an about-face that advocates say was a response to the badgering the Indian government was enduring on all sides.[57]

Across the globe, the pharmaceutical industry keeps a close eye on any proposal that may interfere with its patent monopolies. When a threat is identified, the industry strikes. Pharmaceutical corporations vigorously opposed an indefinite extension at the World Trade Organization of exemptions from medicine patent rules for the poorest countries, lobbied hard against a proposed World Health Organization agreement to support medical research and development, and spent over $126 million resisting a California initiative that would have required drug cost transparency.[58] In opposition to proposals to allow the Medicare program to negotiate drug prices, pharma corporations have published newspaper ads that portray a concerned elderly woman being told "you could lose access to medicines you need."[59] As the National Association of Medicaid Directors said in 2015, "The pharmaceutical industry is the third rail of politics and if you go against them they will cut you off at the knees."[60]

The industry even harshly criticized the TPP measure that would have created the controversial mandate of data exclusivity for biologic drugs. The TPP provisions represented a historic extension of monopoly medicine rights, but the companies wanted even more, complaining that the additional monopoly period of five to eight years was not long enough.[61] These are all quite public efforts, but the pharmaceutical corporations do not limit themselves to above-ground advocacy. As I have discussed (chapter 4), the industry funds patient groups that then lobby for extended patents. Sometimes, large corporations simply buy the generic companies that otherwise might have offered more affordable medicines.[62]

Yet, try as they might, pharmaceutical corporations have not been able to silence the voices of the access-to-medicine advocates. That was certainly true in the historic turn-of-the-twenty-first-century HIV/AIDS treatment campaign, and it has been the case ever since. There are several examples from which activists can draw inspiration:

- In 2007, when the U.S. government and the drug corporation Abbott resisted plans by the Thai government to allow the manufacturing of generic second-line ARV drugs to treat HIV/AIDS, advocacy groups pushed back harder, including a threat to boycott Abbott products. The company eventually dropped its patented price to below the generic price.[63] Thai activists also persuaded their government to create a national HIV/AIDS treatment plan, helped scuttle a proposed United States-Thailand trade agreement that would have included damaging medicine patent protections, and convinced their government to allow the manufacturing of four patented cancer medicines in generic form.[64]
- Activists in Chile have resisted patent-sheltering trade deals and successfully pushed for a Congressional resolution demanding generic licensing of essential medicines.[65]
- Following up on the dramatically successful campaign that led to the dismissal of the pharmaceutical industry lawsuit in 2001, South Africans continued to use civil disobedience, mass protests, and litigation to force the pharmaceutical corporations to allow the generic manufacture of affordable HIV/AIDS medicines.[66]
- Colombian activists have won Congressional endorsement for their demands for generic cancer medicines, and a Kenyan coalition persuaded its parliament to allow greater generic drug access.[67]

- Court victories that expanded medicine access, usually buttressed by significant advocacy outside the legal system, have been won in Peru, Argentina, Venezuela, Colombia, Costa Rica, and Kenya.[68] A study of over 1,000 access-to-medicine lawsuits filed in southern Brazil found that the litigation served as an effective grassroots tool for the poor.[69]

A recent and powerful advocacy success story can be found in the spirited responses by global activists to the prospect of a sweeping pro-patent Trans-Pacific Partnership Agreement.[70] In 2013, José Luis Silva, then the trade minister of Peru, responding to activist outrage, said that proposed intellectual property terms, especially medicine patent rules, elevated the interests of U.S. corporations over the needs of Peruvian citizens. Silva called for Peru to "not go one millimeter beyond what was already negotiated" on medicine access issues in past agreements.[71] Australian access-to-medicine organizations pushed their government to publicly promise that no TPP provisions were acceptable if they undermined the popular pharmaceutical price control program of the country.[72] The Malaysian prime minister condemned any trade agreement restrictions on government efforts to provide affordable medicine as "imping(ing) on fundamentally the sovereign right of the country to make regulation and policy."[73]Similar TPP concerns were expressed by current or former officials in Singapore, New Zealand, Chile, and Canada.[74]

It turns out that all these public statements were the reflection of a dynamic that was being played out even more intensely in the private TPP negotiations. Multiple individuals familiar with the five-plus years of negotiations confirmed that the U.S. proposals to extend medicine monopolies had been opposed by nearly all the other participating nations, with the sometimes exception of Japan.[75]The U.S. publication *Politico* reported that the draft TPP intellectual property chapter as of May 11, 2015, was a ninety-page document "cluttered with objections from other TPP nations" to U.S.-drafted protections for pharmaceutical companies.[76] Negotiators from the TPP nations besides the U.S., supported by global health activists, pushed back hard against extensions to monopoly patent protections.[77]

The result of this resistance was that the U.S. and the pharmaceutical industry, accustomed to getting their way with pro-patent provisions in prior trade agreements, could not achieve their TPP goal of twelve years of data exclusivity for monopoly protection for biologic drugs, forcing an industry-resisted compromise of five to eight years of data exclusivity.[78]

Even with that concession to access-to-medicine arguments, the agreement signed in 2015 by trade ministers still faced real difficulties in getting the necessary legislative approval in several countries, including the United States[79] Ultimately, the deal collapsed in January 2017, when newly-elected U.S. President Donald Trump formally withdrew from the agreement.[80] Many problematic aspects of the TPP spurred determined global opposition, including provisions that would have been harmful for workers and the environment.[81] But the TPP's demise was caused in significant part by what one account called "a small, international group of affordable-medicine advocates" that relentlessly demonstrated in the streets, recruited expert and politically-powerful opposition to the deal, and traveled the globe to button-hole the TPP negotiators and elected officials.[82]

The United States, despite being home to the government that pushes the medicine monopoly agenda on the world stage, is also the site of a growing medicines-access advocacy movement. Accounts of the U.S. withdrawal from the TPP said the agreement had become "politically toxic" for members of both major political parties in the United States, a toxicity medicines-access advocates helped create.[83] When the Obama administration argued for historic levels of intellectual property protection at the TPP negotiating table, U.S.-based economists, elected officials, and presidential candidates, all informed by activist research and fueled by activist demonstrations, raised their voices in opposition to the TPP.[84] The powerful AARP (formerly the American Association of Retired Persons) and the largest U.S. nurses' union were among many health organizations in the United States arguing that TPP provisions could have limited future efforts to control domestic drug prices in programs such as Medicare and Medicaid.[85]

The AARP, along with the California Nurses Association, also supported the November 2016 California ballot initiative designed to lower the prices that the state agencies pay for medicine, one of several state-level initiatives whose aim was reducing drug prices.[86] The California proposal, which was ultimately defeated after the pharmaceutical industry devoted $126 million to campaign against it, called for state agencies to pay no more for medicines than the cost paid by the U.S. Veterans Administration. (The ability of the Veterans Administration to negotiate the prices it pays for the drugs it purchases and to restrict its formulary, freedoms denied the Medicare program, have led to the administration paying an estimated 40 percent less for drugs than Medicare plans do.[87])

Other activism has come in response to the high price set by Gilead for its hepatitis C medicines, including a "Gilead Greed Kills!" advocacy campaign. That campaign conducted demonstrations in front of the company headquarters in Foster City, California, highlighted by a hearse and a plane flying overhead with the campaign message.[88] This kind of activism, along with lawsuits and media coverage, have led to increased government and private-insurer coverage of the hepatitis C medicines, despite their enormous expense.[89]

During the 2016 Democratic and Republican Party conventions, access-to-medicine activists staged a mock tug-of-war and took out full-page newspaper ads featuring a character named Big Pharma Bro; the aim was to demonstrate the overall support of the pharmaceutical corporate agenda by both parties.[90] I have already mentioned (chapters 2 and 4) that the 450 percent increase in the price of the allergy shot EpiPen, a product that enjoyed a market monopoly, triggered what *USA Today* called a "firestorm" of controversy and angry condemnations from lawmakers and patients.[91] Access-to-medicine advocates have disrupted congressional hearings, filed U.S. lawsuits, sent public letters decrying the prices of patented medicines, and supported local and state initiatives demanding negotiated drug prices and cost transparency.[92]

Healthcare providers often play important roles in that advocacy. In 2016, a physician wrote a column in the *Los Angeles Times* that began, "The drug companies are ripping us off, pill by pill, shot by shot. Instead of working to earn reasonable returns by relieving our suffering and saving lives, they now focus on profits above all."[93] That same year, another physician wrote in the *Salt Lake Tribune*, "Evil in medicine is often linked with the past practices of blood-letting, lobotomies and arsenic treatments. Now we can add to these atrocities another evil, that of killing people by preventing their needed, life-sustaining treatments."[94]

Faith-based groups are advancing a similarly morality-based argument against medicine monopoly pricing. "The field is tilted toward the powers that be rather than the power of God's people," stated one coalition letter in opposition to the TPP. "Our faith organizations serve those living in poverty in every country in the world and stand witness to the pain that bad trade policies inflict on communities, particularly developing

countries."[95] An interfaith investor coalition is pushing shareholder resolutions to force the pharma corporations to justify their price increases.[96]
In recognition of the key role that faith-based organizations have played
in recent successful social movements, including the U.S. civil rights and
labor movements, I am part of a group that has launched an effort to
advance this faith community advocacy; our organization is called People
of Faith for Access to Medicines (PFAM).[97]

As was the case with the HIV/AIDS treatment campaign, recent access-to-
medicines activism has featured leading roles played by affected patients.
Manon Ress and Phillipa Saunders, breast cancer patients and members of
the Union for Affordable Cancer Treatment, were instrumental in pushing
the UK government to allow the generic manufacturing of the breast cancer drug T-DM1, actions that eventually forced the patent-holder Roche
to lower its price.[98] Cancer patients holding an IV pole that read "TPP:
Don't Cut My IV" disrupted TPP negotiations in 2015 and, as we have
learned (chapter 1), were arrested protesting at PhRMA headquarters on
World Cancer Day in 2016.[99] One of those patients, Zahara Heckscher,
is a U.S. resident and has been treated with patented biologic drugs that
would have been subject to extended monopoly protection and unaffordable pricing under TPP. "One of my current cancer medicines could cost
me over $100,000 if I were not in a clinical trial," Hecksher told the
media after her arrest. "If [the TPP] passes, thousands of women like me
will die waiting."[100]

Some patients are taking affordable access to medicine into their own
hands. Lu Yong, a Chinese leukemia patient, violated national law by
purchasing and distributing generic medicines from India to his fellow
patients. When Yong faced charges for his actions, hundreds of those Chinese leukemia patients petitioned the court on his behalf. Their advocacy
seemed to have an impact; soon after the patients' petition was filed, the
Chinese patent office invalidated the national patent on the medicines that
Yong was importing.[101]

Greg Jefferys, a hepatitis C patient in Australia, similarly has openly
broken the law by importing generic medicines for fellow patients, including patients in the United States "The patients with liver cirrhosis are
sitting there and waiting," Jeffreys said. "And so I'd have to ask the
(patent-holding) company—how do you sleep at night?"[102]

In India, patient groups are currently pushing hard for access to affordable breast cancer and hepatitis C drugs. Their efforts follow in the footsteps of Indian patients who helped lead a very successful 2005–2013 campaign for access to a leukemia treatment.[103] It is a campaign that is worth reviewing here, as it holds several promising lessons for current activists.

The leukemia treatment in question was imatinib mesylate, the most effective medicine for chronic myeloid leukemia. The pharmaceutical corporation Novartis holds patents on the medicine, which it markets as Glivec or Gleevec. When its original Indian patent on the drug was running out, Novartis applied to patent a new form of the medicine, this one in beta crystalline form, thus extending its monopoly.

In response, a generic manufacturer and the Cancer Patients Aid Association (CPAA) opposed the patent application, charging Novartis with pursuing a classic evergreening effort; that is, the company was trying to prolong its patent by introducing a new version of the drug that was not significantly different, much less better, than the original.[104] For Indians with leukemia, the stakes were life and death. The generic version of imatinib mesylate was priced at $170 per month, while patent-protected Glivec sold in some countries for as much as $3,000 per month, far out of the reach of most Indian leukemia patients.[105]

In January 2006, the Indian Patents Office refused the Novartis application, agreeing with the challengers that the new version of the drug was not a significant innovation on the older version.[106] Novartis filed an appeal. Anand Grover, a distinguished Indian lawyer who was also serving as the UN special rapporteur on the right to health, signed on to represent the CPAA. As years of appeals dragged on, the CPAA showed real staying power, sticking with the case in the face of both threats and offers of cash from Novartis.[107]

The struggle was intense, in both India and beyond. Novartis recruited U.S. government officials to exert trade pressure on India, while Indian activists and attorneys mobilized in the courts and in the streets.[108] When the case was argued before judges, advocates conducted loud demonstrations outside the courthouse.[109] Indian activists were joined by international organizations such as Médecins Sans Frontières/Doctors Without Borders (MSF) and Knowledge Ecology International. MSF organized a 2006 Drop the Case campaign against Novartis, circulating a petition signed by nearly a half million people, and conducted a global day of action on the eve of a 2012 Novartis board meeting.[110] Activists persuaded Dr. Brian Druker, whose research had helped develop imatinib mesylate, to write an open letter urging broader access to the medicine.[111]

Finally, on April 1, 2013, the Supreme Court of India issued a final rejection of the Novartis patent claim. The court wrote a strongly worded anti-evergreening decision that underscored that Indian law does not allow monopoly extensions based on minor drug changes that do not add therapeutic value.[112]

A dozen years after the dramatic success of the HIV/AIDS treatment campaign, access-to-medicine activists had won another huge victory. The time is right to lay the groundwork for the next one.

I have now spent many pages discussing how patients suffer without medicines, how pharmaceutical corporations make enormous monopoly profits, and how a money-corrupted system produces this injustice. By now, I hope you are asking, "What can I do to make this change?" Inspired by the dedicated access-to-medicine activists around the world, from South Africa to India to the United States, here are some answers to that question.

Join an Existing Access-to-Medicines Team

You are now well aware that there are several organizations filled with dedicated and knowledgeable activists working hard to increase access to medicines. The globally admired MSF conducts an access-to-medicines campaign that includes public education about the corrupted system and direct calls for advocacy on issues such as vaccine pricing.[113] Sometimes MSF-led activism calls for contacting lawmakers on issues such as the TPP; sometimes it is more creative. For example, in late 2015, MSF activists dumped $17 million in fake cash at the New York City headquarters of Pfizer, representing the daily revenue that the company makes on vaccine sales.[114] Those efforts are bearing fruit: in late 2016, MSF advocates achieved a significant victory when the two manufacturers of the vaccine against the leading cause of pneumonia agreed to reduce the price they charge to humanitarian organizations, a corporate change of heart that MSF attributed to advocates' petitions, calls, tweets, and in-person demonstrations.[115]

Several other advocacy groups also do great work. Knowledge Ecology International is known for its mastery of the complex details of the laws and trade terms that impact access to medicines.[116] U.S.-based Public Citizen leverages the size and reputation of a broad-based consumer action organization to call for access to medicines.[117] I have discussed the student-led group Universities Allied for Essential Medicines (chapter 21), which has recruited prominent members of the international scientific and academic communities to push for a global medicines research agreement to fund research and require that medicines be available at affordable prices.[118] I have also mentioned a new organization I am involved in, People of Faith for Access to Medicines, which has the aim of building a faith community base for access-to-medicines advocacy.[119]

All these organizations would love your help at whatever level of involvement you can take on, ranging from starting a local, congregation, or campus chapter to simply retweeting and sharing their regular calls to sign petitions, share your story, and push lawmakers. Check their websites for more about how you can pitch in.

Another action opportunity for you is to reach out to the organization or community ties you already have and urge them to make access-to-medicines activism a top item on their agenda. As we have learned, faith-based organizations, the AARP, and unions all have lent their voices to the access-to-medicines cause. But those voices will be louder and more insistent with your help. This is especially true if you are a health care provider; when organizations such as the California Nurses Association, Physicians for a National Health Program, and the American Medical Association speak out demanding reform in the medicines system, their voices carry great weight.[120]

Access-to-medicines activists know well that they are facing a formidable challenge. But James Love, the legendary founder of Knowledge Ecology International, is one of many who express real optimism for the cause. "I don't think [the pharmaceutical companies] are all-powerful. I think a rag-tag group of activists are stronger," Love said. "The American people do care. They agree with us, not Big Pharma."[121]

Create Your Own Access-to-Medicines Team

Chances are that you or a loved one has faced the frightening experience of needing medicines to alleviate suffering or even save a life. Being sick or being in support of someone who is can produce a feeling of helplessness. But that difficult experience also provides insights, credibility, and impact for an access-to-medicines activist. The HIV/AIDS treatment movement has demonstrated the power of patients and their loved ones pushing for medicines reform. Patients such as Hannah Lyon, whom we met in chapter 1 at the beginning of this book, are proving that model can still work today. She and fellow cancer patient Zahara Heckscher created Cancer Families for Affordable Medicines, and their new organization is already an effective force for the human right to essential medicines.[122] So are Patients for Affordable Drugs and T1 International, which provide passionate and uncompromising patient voices.[123]

Tell Your Elected Officials about Access to Medicines

Elected officials at every level have enormous influence on the availability and prices of medicines. As we have discussed, government decisions fuel medicines research, write the rules that create monopoly patents, and divert billions of taxpayer dollars to pharmaceutical corporations. Those corporations know well how much power elected officials have over the medicines process, which is why they employ thousands of lobbyists and direct hundreds of millions of dollars each year to lobbying and campaign contributions. Our elected officials hear plenty from Big Pharma; they need to hear from patients and taxpayers, too.

Because I am a U.S. law professor writing a book for a U.S. publisher, it is very likely that you are a reader from the United States. If so, that means you have a great opportunity. The U.S. government that represents us is far and away the most influential player in the medicines system. Our elected officials are the ones who pass the laws that protect corporate monopolies and guarantee that we have the highest prices for medicines in the world. Our elected officials are the ones using trade deals to pressure other governments to give corporations the power to push up medicine prices around the world. If the United States exercises its right to withdraw from these trade deals, as other nations have recently done in response to the required Investor-State Dispute Systems provision, or rejects a deal such as the TPP outright, as it did in January 2017, those actions have an enormous global impact.[124] The current profits-over-people medicine system is in large part a U.S. creation, so U.S. elected officials—spurred on by your and my activism—need to play a role in dismantling it.

Tell Your Friends, Family, Classmates, and Coworkers about Access to Medicines

As we have seen, a large majority of Americans feel that drug prices are unreasonable and that drug companies are putting profits before people.[125] That provides a good platform for our activism; studies of social movements show that frustration is a precondition for social change. But most of those angry people do not know why our medicines system is so broken or what can be done to fix it. Those same studies of social movements show that frustration leads to change only when the cause of the problem is properly labeled and a clear alternative is presented.[126]

That is where you come in. Person by person, you can help label the problem and identify the solution. You can explain how medicines do not have to be expensive and unattainable, and you can help transform that frustration into action.

While it would be nice if you could convince your skeptical roommate or your belligerent Uncle Earl to read the preceding twenty-two chapters in this book—and to peruse the hundreds of endnotes as well—that is usually not a realistic plan. Most of the time, we are players in a Short-Attention-Span Theater. So, here are a few talking points you can use when discussing access to medicines, along with references to the chapters in this book to bolster your point. If you connect with an access-to-medicines organization, which I recommend you do, the organization will regularly provide specific messages and suggested targets for those messages. But these talking points will give you the big-picture arguments.

"Taxpayers are paying twice for medicines" (chapter 15). There are few more potent calls to action than telling taxpayers they are getting ripped off. With medicines, that charge is absolutely true. Taxpayers pay to support the most important drug research, only to have government officials hand over the fruits of that research as monopoly patents to corporations. Then, the corporations turn around and charge enormous prices to those same taxpayers, through out-of-pocket payments; insurance premiums; or costs billed to Medicare, Medicaid, or the Veterans Administration. This has to stop.

"Medicine patents stifle innovation. Open-source development would lead to lifesaving improvements" (chapters 12 and 13). This may be an especially important point to make to younger, tech-savvy individuals who appreciate the wonderful developments made possible by the open software movement. The patent system is great for generating monopoly profits, but its secrecy and exclusivity has proven to block new inventions. Ask your listeners to imagine what amazing treatments could be developed if medicine researchers were unleashed to build on the existing medicine knowledge that the patent system is locking away.

"The medicines system is the very opposite of a free-market system; corporations rely on government-provided monopolies that block competition and allow them to charge artificially inflated prices" (chapters 12, 18, and 19). Your Uncle Earl is likely to be a fan of the free market system—most Americans are. So it is important to point out that the massive financial success of pharmaceutical corporations spits in the face of free market principles.

Not only do these corporations rely on government-granted monopolies and avoid fair competition like the plague, they lean on government to make the riskiest investments in early-stage medicines research. In the pharmaceutical industry, the risks are socialized, but the rewards are privatized. Similarly, when it comes to medicines, the so-called "free trade" agreements are not about free trade at all. Patents are nothing if not competition-blocking protectionism, and medicine monopolies are estimated to equate to a whopping 10,000 percent tariff.[127]

"Medicine prices are not high because of research costs; they are high because of windfall profits and wasteful advertising" (chapters 7 and 10). When it comes to the reasons for high medicine prices, do not let your friends and family buy what Big Pharma is selling. Sky-high price tags at the pharmacy are funding endless erectile dysfunction drug ads—which your Uncle Earl is no doubt tired of watching on TV because they interrupt his football games. Americans pay the highest medicine prices in the world to fund those commercials, along with high-volume lobbying and marketing to lawmakers and physicians, not to mention record-setting profit margins. The high prices do *not* fund medicine research. Which leads to the next talking point:

"We can change this system immediately because governments and nonprofits are already driving the important medicine research" (chapters 9, 20, and 21). We do not have to choose between affordable prices for medicine and aggressive medicine research. Because governments are already funding the most important research now, we can cut costs immediately and substantially. We can do so by eliminating the corporate monopolies that force patients (and the governments that administer the health care programs that so many rely on) to pay for advertising, lobbying, and huge profits. This talking point embraces the critical four-word core of any argument for social change: We. Can. Do. Better.

"Access to medicines is a moral imperative and a human right" (chapters 3, 4, 18, 19, and 22). There is no need to sugar-coat this reality: every day, people are suffering and dying by the thousands simply because the medicines that would help them are priced too high. Corporate profits are taking precedence over the lives of children and young mothers. Tobeka Daki should not have died. Ahmed should not have died.

I bet your listeners will not be comfortable with that deaths-for-profits trade-off. People were not OK with it during the HIV/AIDS crisis in the 1990s and 2000s, when activism-generated outrage turned around the treatment landscape. It shocked our conscience that millions were dying from treatable HIV/AIDS. Today, it is just as appalling that millions die from treatable cancer, or because they could not afford vaccines.

This leads to my concluding point in this book: access-to-medicines advocacy can work. We know that because it already has—both in the HIV/AIDS treatment struggle and in more recent campaigns. It is not going to be easy, of course. But there is a lot of reason for optimism. This is no longer just a struggle being waged by the desperate poor and sick in the developing world and by the caregivers and activists that work with them. Now, as we have seen, these advocates have been joined in their struggle by comparatively wealthy people in richer nations because even these people and their governments cannot pay for the medicine they need. Medicines activists are now joined by frustrated physicians, elected officials, economists, and even hospitals and insurance companies, all calling for a change to this broken system.[128]

And, I hope, they will be joined by you, too. Together, we can cure our sick medicines system.

NOTES

Introduction

1. Ashley Kirzinger, Bryan Wu, and Mollyann Brodie, "Kaiser Health Tracking Poll: September 2016," Kaiser Family Foundation, http://kff.org/report-section/kaiser-health-tracking-poll-september-2016-politics-and-rx-costs/ (last modified September 29, 2016).

2. James Love, interviewed by the author, September 15, 2015.

1. People Everywhere Are Struggling to Get the Medicines They Need

1. I first told Hannah Lyon's story in Fran Quigley, "From Cancer Patient to Medicines Activist," Counterpunch, May 10, 2016, http://www.counterpunch.org/2016/05/10/from-cancer-patient-to-medicines-activist/.

2. Public Citizen Global Trade Watch, "Cancer Patients Arrested at World Cancer Day Protest," YouTube, video, 2:37, February 6, 2016, https://www.youtube.com/watch?v=Els7c-DLdIc.

3. "Sign the Petition for Affordable Medicines," Cancer Families for Affordable Medicine, 2016, http://cancerfam.org/ (accessed June 5, 2016).

4. Jake Harper, "Indiana ACLU Sues to Demand Medicaid Reimburse for Hepatitis C Drugs," Side Effects: Public Media, December 8, 2015, http://sideeffectspublicmedia.org/post/indiana-aclu-sues-demand-medicaid-reimburse-hepatitis-c-drugs; Sarah Jackson et al. v. Secretary of the Indiana Family and Social Services Administration, No. 1:15-cv-01874 (S.D. Ind. filed Nov. 25, 2015). Full disclosure: the author served for a period of time as co-counsel for Ms. Jackson in her suit, and also a proposed class action, to secure access to the prescribed

medicine under the Indiana Medicaid program. All the information discussed here is in the public record, and none of it is privileged information.

5. Organization for Economic Co-Operation and Development, Focus on Health Spending: OECD Health Statistics 2015, 2015, http://www.oecd.org/health/health-systems/Focus-Health-Spending-2015.pdf.

6. Deena Beasley, "Gilead to Raise Price for New Hepatitis C Drug above $84,00," Reuters, September 12, 2014, http://www.reuters.com/article/us-gilead-sovaldi-idUSKBN0H72KR20140912.

7. Gabriel Levitt, "Will Your Private Health Insurance Cover Sovaldi? (Part 2)," PharmacyChecker (blog), September 12, 2014, https://www.pharmacycheckerblog.com/will-your-private-health-insurance-cover-sovaldi-part-2; Dennis Wagner, "VA to Outsource Care for 180,000 Vets with Hepatitis C," Arizona Republic, June 19, 2015, http://www.azcentral.com/story/news/arizona/investigations/2015/06/19/va-outsource-care-vets-hepatitis/28969411/.

8. Soumitri Barua, Robert Greenwald, Jason Grebely, Gregory J. Dore, Tracy Swan, and Lynn E. Taylor, "Restrictions for Medicaid Reimbursement of Sofosbuvir for the Treatment of Hepatitis C Virus Infection in the United States," Annals of Internal Medicine 163, no. 3 (2015): 215–33, doi:10.7326/M15-0406.

9. Orrin G. Hatch and Ron Wyden, Committee on Finance, U.S. Senate, "The Price of Solvadi and Its Impact on the U.S. Health Care System," S. Rep. 114–20 (2015).

10. Swathi Iyengar, Kiu Tay-Teo, Sabine Vogler, Peter Beyer, Stefan Wiktor, Kees de Joncheere, and Suzanne Hill, "Prices, Costs, and Affordability of New Medicines for Hepatitis C in 30 Countries: An Economic Analysis," PLoS Medicine 13, no. 5 (2016): e1002032, http://journals.plos.org/plosmedicine/article?id=10.1371/journal.pmed.1002032.

11. Quoted in Harper, "Indiana ACLU."

12. Public Citizen, "Government Action Needed to Slash Prices for Hepatitis C Treatments: Public Citizen Testifies before the U.S. Committee on Veterans' Affairs, Explains How to Reduce Cost of Therapies," news release, December 3, 2014, http://www.citizen.org/pressroom/pressroomredirect.cfm?ID=4342.

13. Abby Goodnough, "Costly to Treat, Hepatitis C Gains Quietly in U.S.," New York Times, July 23, 2015, http://www.nytimes.com/2015/07/24/us/kentucky-struggles-to-contain-hepatitis-c-among-young-drug-users.html?_r=1.

14. Wagner, "VA to Outsource."

15. Harper, "Indiana ACLU." The medicine has been rationed in England as well; Sarah Bosely, "NHS 'Abandoning' Thousands by Rationing Hepatitis C Drugs," Guardian, July 27, 2016, https://www.theguardian.com/society/2016/jul/28/nhs-abandoning-thousands-by-rationing-hepatitis-c-drugs?CMP=share_btn_tw.

16. Centers for Disease Control and Prevention, "Viral Hepatitis—Hepatitis C Information," last modified January 8, 2016, http://www.cdc.gov/hepatitis/hcv/cfaq.htm#overview; Centers for Disease Control and Prevention, "Hepatitis FAQ's for Health Professionals," last modified March 11, 2016, http://www.cdc.gov/hepatitis/hcv/hcvfaq.htm.

17. World Health Organization, "Hepatitis C," last modified July, 2016, http://www.who.int/mediacentre/factsheets/fs164/en/.

18. Chloé Forette, "Defuse Hepatitis C, the Viral Time Bomb: Test and Treat Hepatitis C," paper presented at the 67th World Health Assembly, Geneva, May 2014, http://www.hepcoalition.org/advocate/advocacy-tools/article/defuse-hepatitis-c-the-viral-time.

19. Jon E. Zibbell, Kashif Iqbal, Rajiv C. Patel, Anil Suryaprasad, Kathy J. Sanders, Loretta Moore-Moravian, Jamie Serrecchia, Steven Blankenship, John W. Ward, and Deborah Holtzman, "Increases in Hepatitis C Virus Infection Related to Injection Drug Use among Persons Aged ≤30 Years—Kentucky, Tennessee, Virginia, and West Virginia, 2006–2012," Morbidity and Mortality Weekly Report 64, no. 17 (2015): 453–58, http://www.cdc.gov/mmwr/preview/mmwrhtml/mm6417a2.htm.

20. Richard Martinello and David Ross, State of Care for Veterans with Hepatitis C (Washington, DC: U.S. Department of Veterans Affairs, 2014), http://www.hepatitis.va.gov/pdf/HCV-State-of-Care-2014.pdf.

21. Liz Highleyman, "EASL 2014: Sofosbuvir + Ledipasvir Cures More than 90% of First-Time and Retreated Genotype 1 Patients," HIVandHepatitis.com, April 12, 2014, http://www.hivandhepatitis.com/hcv-treatment/experimental-hcv-drugs/4627-easl-2014-sofosbuvirledipasvir-cures-more-than-90-of-first-time-and-retreated-genotype-1-patients.

22. Andrew Hill, Saye Khoo, Joe Fortunak, Bryony Simmons, and Nathan Ford, "Minimum Costs for Producing Hepatitis C Direct-Acting Antivirals for Use in Large-Scale Treatment Access Programs in Developing Countries," Clinical Infectious Diseases 58 2014): 928–36, doi: 10.1093/cid/ciu012.

23. Eric Pianin, "Costly Hepatitis 'C' Drug Makers Face New Fire," Fiscal Times, December 4, 2014, http://www.thefiscaltimes.com/2014/12/04/Costly-Hepatitis-C-Drug-Makers-Face-New-Fire; Ed Silverman, "Gilead Is Accused of Price Gouging, but Is There Really a Legal Argument?" Pharmalot (blog), Wall Street Journal, December 19, 2014, http://blogs.wsj.com/pharmalot/2014/12/19/gilead-is-accused-of-price-gouging-but-is-there-really-a-legal-argument/; Maggie Flick and Ben Hirschler, "Gilead Offers Egypt New Hepatitis C Drug at 99 Percent Discount," Reuters, March 21, 2014, http://www.reuters.com/article/us-hepatitis-egypt-gilead-sciences-idUSBREA2K1VF20140321.

24. Médecins Sans Frontières/Doctors Without Borders, "Gilead's Chronic Hepatitis C Treatment Expansion Restrictions: Committed to Limiting Access to Affordable Generic Medicines for Millions of People Who Can Benefit from Them in Developing Countries," modified March 2015, http://www.msfaccess.org/sites/default/files/MSF_assets/HepC/Docs/HepC_factsheet_GileadHCVTreatmentRestriction_BNG_2015.pdf.

25. Susan Heavey, "U.S. Drug Industry Group Defends Price of Gilead Hepatitis Drug," Reuters, April 10, 2014, http://www.reuters.com/article/us-hepatitis-gilead-phrma-idUSBREA3911220140410.

26. Jeffrey Sachs, "The Drug That Is Bankrupting America," Huffington Post (blog), February 16, 2015, http://www.huffingtonpost.com/jeffrey-sachs/the-drug-that-is-bankrupt_b_6692340.html. Veronika J. Wirtz, Hans V. Hogerzeil, Andrew L. Gray, Maryam Bigdeli, Cornelis P. de Joncheere, Margaret A. Ewen, Martha Gyansa-Lutterodt, Sun Jing, Vera L Luiza, Regina M Mbindyo, Helene Möller, Corrina Moucheraud, Bernard Pécoul, Lembit Rägo, Arash Rashidian, Dennis Ross-Degnan, Peter N. Stephens, Yot Teerawattananon, Ellen F. M. 't Hoen, Anita K Wagner, Prashant Yadav, Michael R. Reich, "Essential Medicines for Universal Health Coverage," The Lancet, November 7, 2016, http://yolse.org/wp-content/uploads/2016/11/EssentialMeds.pdf, 16.

27. Eduardo Porter, "Government R&D, Private Profits and the American Taxpayer," New York Times, May 26, 2015, http://www.nytimes.com/2015/05/27/business/giving-taxpayers-a-cut-when-government-rd-pays-off-for-industry.html.

2. The United States Has a Drug Problem

1. Center for Responsive Politics, "Top Industries: Lobbying," last modified August 2015, https://www.opensecrets.org/lobby/top.php?indexType=i; Diane Archer, "Strengthen Medicare: End Drug Company Price Setting," Health Affairs (blog), May 28, 2013, http://healthaffairs.org/blog/2013/05/28/strengthen-medicare-end-drug-company-price-setting/.

2. "Sales of Sovaldi, New Gilead Hepatitis C Drug, Soar to $10.3 Billion," New York Times, February 3, 2015, http://www.nytimes.com/2015/02/04/business/sales-of-sovaldi-new-gilead-hepatitis-c-drug-soar-to-10-3-billion.html; Jeffrey Sachs, "Gilead's Greed That Kills," Huffington Post (blog), July 27, 2015, http://www.huffingtonpost.com/jeffrey-sachs/gileads-greed-that-kills_b_7878102.html.

3. Gary Strauss, "Gilead Sciences CEO Martin: $180 Million Man," USA Today, March 15, 2014, http://www.usatoday.com/story/money/markets/2014/03/14/gilead-sciences-ceo-cashes-inagain/6430209/.

4. Karen Ignagni, "We All Pay for $1,000 a Pill Drug," Opinion: Political Op-Eds, CNN, July 24, 2014, http://www.cnn.com/2014/07/07/opinion/ignagni-hepatitis-c-drug/.

5. Michelle Andrews, "People with Diabetes Are Facing Rising Prices for Lifesaving Drugs," Washington Post, August 24, 2015, http://www.washingtonpost.com/national/health-science/people-with-diabetes-are-facing-rising-prices-for-lifesaving-drugs/2015/08/24/dec2abd8-476f-11e5-8e7d-9c033e6745d8_story.html.

6. Kasia Lipska, "Break Up the Insulin Racket," New York Times, February 20, 2016, http://www.nytimes.com/2016/02/21/opinion/sunday/break-up-the-insulin-racket.html.

7. Ibid.; quoted in Alan Jude Ryland, "The Epipen Wasn't Alone: Price Gouging On Insulin Draws Outrage," Second Nexus, September 16, 2016, http://secondnexus.com/social-commentary-and-trends/price-gouging-on-insulin/?utm_content=inf_10_1164_2&tse_id=IN F_672767707c1211e6bf8e470556fe0b22.

8. Lipska, "Break Up the Insulin Racket"; Andrews, "People "People with Diabetes."

9. Donald Chaires, George Denault, Jane Doe, John Doe, Brittany Gilleland, Gerald Girard, Sara Hasselbach, Lindsey Kinhan, Joseph Mclaughlin, Matthew Teachman, and Karyn Wofford, Plaintiffs, v. Sanofi U.S., Novo Nordisk Inc., and Eli Lilly and Company, Class Action Complaint Filed January 30, 2017, 7, U.S. District Court of Massachusetts, No. 1:17-cv-10158, https://www.hbsslaw.com/uploads/case_downloads/insulin/01-30-17_insulin_class_action_complaint_hagens_berman.pdf.

10. James Elliott, telephone interview with the author, February 27, 2017.

11. Andrew Pollack, "Drug Goes from $13.50 a Tablet to $750, Overnight," New York Times, September 20, 2015, http://www.nytimes.com/2015/09/21/business/a-huge-overnight-increase-in-a-drugs-price-raises-protests.html (regarding heart disease, tuberculosis, and anti-biotics); Andrew Pollack, "New Cholesterol Drugs Are Vastly Overpriced, Analysis Says," New York Times, September 8, 2015, http://www.nytimes.com/2015/09/09/business/new-cholesterol-drugs-are-vastly-overpriced-analysis-says.html (regarding high cholesterol).

12. Elizabeth Rosenthal, "The Price of Prevention: Vaccine Costs Are Soaring," New York Times, July 2, 2014, http://www.nytimes.com/2014/07/03/health/Vaccine-Costs-Soaring-Paying-Till-It-Hurts.html?_r=0.

13. Pollack, "Drug Goes from $13.50."

14. Nathan Bomey, "EpiPen Maker to Offer Discounts after Price Hike Firestorm," USA Today, August 26, 2016, http://www.usatoday.com/story/money/2016/08/25/epipen-maker-offer-discounts-after-firestorm/89329122/.

15. Jonathan D. Rockoff, "Rising Drug Costs to Be in Focus at Congressional Hearing: Valeant, Turing Pharmaceuticals and Other Companies Have Been under Fire over Rising Drug Prices," Wall Street Journal, December 5, 2015, http://www.wsj.com/articles/rising-drug-costs-to-be-in-focus-at-congressional-hearing-1449311407; Paul Demko and Sarah Karlin, "GOP Candidates Stuck on Drug Prices," Politico, December 1, 2015, http://www.politico.com/story/2015/11/drug-costs-gop-candidates-prescriptions-216292.

16. Cynthia Koons, "Pfizer Raised Prices on 133 Drugs This Year, and It's Not Alone," Bloomberg News, October 2, 2015, http://www.bloomberg.com/news/articles/2015-10-02/pfizer-raised-prices-on-133-drugs-this-year-and-it-s-not-alone; "U.S. Inflation Calculator: Historical Inflation Rates: 1914–2016," Coin News Media Group, http://www.usinflationcalculator.com/inflation/historical-inflation-rates/ (accessed May 13, 2016); Brady Dennis, "Prescription Drug Prices Jump More than 10 Percent in 2015, Analysis Finds," Washington Post, January 11, 2016, https://www.washingtonpost.com/news/to-your-health/wp/2016/01/11/prescription-drug-prices-jumped-more-than-10-percent-in-2015/; Peter Sullivan, "Sanders to Introduce

Bill Targeting High Drug Prices," The Hill, September 1, 2015, http://thehill.com/policy/healthcare/252473-sanders-to-introduce-bill-targeting-high-drug-prices.

17. "Report Finds Drug Prices Driving Increased Health Care Costs," The Campaign For Sustainable Drug Pricing (blog), May 10, 2016, http://www.csrxp.org/sp-report-finds-rx-prices-driving-increased-health-care-costs/.

18. Carolyn Y. Johnson, "Why America Pays So Much More for Drugs," Washington Post, February 25, 2016, https://www.washingtonpost.com/news/wonk/wp/2016/02/25/why-america-pays-so-much-more-for-drugs/; Aaron S. Kesselheim, Jerry Avorn, and Ameet Sarpatwari, "The High Cost of Prescription Drugs in the United States Origins and Prospects for Reform," Journal of the American Medical Association 316, no. 8 (August 23/30, 2016): 858–71, doi:10.1001/jama.2016.11237.

19. James Love, telephone interview with the author, September 15, 2015.

20. Gregg Gonsalves, "Martin Shkreli Is Just a Tiny Part of a Huge Problem," Nation, September 25, 2015, http://www.thenation.com/article/martin-shkreli-is-just-a-tiny-part-of-a-huge-problem/. Veronika J Wirtz, Hans V Hogerzeil, Andrew L Gray, Maryam Bigdeli, Cornelis P de Joncheere, Margaret A Ewen, Martha Gyansa-Lutterodt, Sun Jing, Vera L Luiza, Regina M Mbindyo, Helene Möller, Corrina Moucheraud, Bernard Pécoul, Lembit Rägo, Arash Rashidian, Dennis Ross-Degnan, Peter N Stephens, Yot Teerawattananon, Ellen F M 't Hoen, Anita K Wagner, Prashant Yadav, Michael R Reich, "Essential Medicines for Universal Health Coverage," The Lancet, November 7, 2016, http://yolse.org/wp-content/uploads/2016/11/EssentialMeds.pdf, 34.

21. David Crow, "Price of Cancer Drugs Vastly Higher in US, According to Study," Financial Times June 6, 2016, https://www.ft.com/content/851cd240-2b6f-11e6-bf8d-26294ad519fc.

22. Drew Altman, "Prescription Drugs' Sizable Share of Health Spending," Washington Wire (blog), Wall Street Journal, December 13, 2015, http://blogs.wsj.com/washwire/2015/12/13/prescription-drugs-sizable-share-of-health-spending/.

23. U.S. Department of Health and Human Services, "Prescription Drugs: Innovation, Spending, and Patient Access," Report to Congress, December 7, 2016, http://apps.who.int/medicinedocs/documents/s23128en/s23128en.pdf, 4; George Underwood, "Global Drug Spend to Reach $1.4 Trillion," Pharma Times, November 18, 2015, http://www.pharma times.com/Article/15-11-18/Global_drug_spend_to_reach_1_4_trillion.aspx.

24. Nick Triggle, "NHS Says No to New Breast Cancer Drug Kadcyla," BBC News, August 8, 2014, http://www.bbc.com/news/health-28688311; "Join the Fix the Patent Laws Campaign," Infojustice.org (blog), American University Program on Information Justice and Intellectual Property, February 5, 2015, http://infojustice.org/archives/33877.

25. Steven Ross Johnson, "CEO Power Panel: Healthcare Leaders Back Feds Stepping in to Restrain Drug Prices," Modern Healthcare, November 14, 2015, http://www.modern healthcare.com/article/20151114/MAGAZINE/311149963.

26. Henry J. Kaiser Family Foundation, "2015 Employer Health Benefits Survey," http://kff.org/report-section/ehbs-2015-summary-of-findings/. Some insurance companies refuse coverage or require onerous copayments for some of the highest-cost drugs; Fran Quigley, "The $100,000 Pill: How U.S. Health Agencies Are Choosing Pharma over Patients," Truthout, August 5, 2016, http://www.truth-out.org/news/item/37111-the-100-000-per-year-pill-how-us-health-agencies-choose-pharma-over-patients; Bill Spencer, "Houston Mother Forced to Pay Triple Price for Cancer Drug after Insurance Company Denies Coverage," Click2Houston, February 9, 2016, http://www.click2houston.com/news/investigates/pa tients-being-forced-to-choose-between-life-money; Sara Hansard, "Prescription Drug Costs 'Number One Driving Factor' for Rising Health Insurance Premiums," BNA Healthcare Blog (blog), Bloomberg, June 30, 2016, http://www.bna.com/prescription-drug-costs-b57982 076322/.

27. Shefali Luthra, "Consumers Still Struggling with Medical Debt," USA Today, February 1, 2015, http://www.usatoday.com/story/news/2015/02/01/consumers-still-struggling-with-medical-debt/22587749/.

28. Alison Kodjak, "Medical Bills Still Take a Big Toll, Even with Insurance," Shots: Health News from NPR, National Public Radio, March 8, 2016, http://www.npr.org/sections/health-shots/2016/03/08/468892489/medical-bills-still-take-a-big-toll-even-with-insurance.

29. Gabriel Levitt, "50 Million Americans, Ages 19–64, Forgo Meds in 2012 Due to Cost; 37% of Seniors Concerned about Drug Prices," PharmacyChecker (blog), PharmacyChecker.com, May 10, 2013, https://www.pharmacycheckerblog.com/50-million-americans-ages-19-64-forgo-meds-in-2012-due-to-cost.

30. U.S. Department of Health and Human Services, "Prescription Drugs: Innovation, Spending, and Patient Access," 102, Report to Congress, December 7, 2016, http://apps.who.int/medicinedocs/documents/s23128en/s23128en.pdf.

31. Sheri Fink, "Drug Shortages Forcing Hard Decisions on Rationing Treatments," New York Times, January 29, 2016, http://www.nytimes.com/2016/01/29/us/drug-shortages-forcing-hard-decisions-on-rationing-treatments.html; Sabrina Tavernise, "Drug Shortages Continue to Vex Doctors," New York Times, February 10, 2014, http://www.nytimes.com/2014/02/11/health/shortages-of-critical-drugs-continue-to-vex-doctors-study-finds.html.

32. Fink, "Drug Shortages."

33. Ibid.

34. Ibid.

35. See, for example, Tavernise, "Drug Shortages Continue to Vex Doctors." (Only three manufacturers produced 71 percent of sterile injectable cancer drugs.)

36. Fink, "Drug Shortages."

37. "What's Behind the Nation's Prescription Drug Shortage?" PBS NewsHour, February 16, 2014, http://www.pbs.org/newshour/bb/whats-behind-nations-prescription-drug-shortage/.

3. Millions of People Are Dying Needlessly

1. Fix the Patent Laws, "South Africa: Access to Critical Breast Cancer Drug Trastuzumab Limited by Patent Laws," YouTube video, 03:59. posted February 2016, https://www.youtube.com/watch?v=Vl5AJa7_pDY&feature=youtu.be. ; Knowledge Ecology International, "Thobeka Daki, on High Price of Herceptin, Lack of Access," YouTube video, 03:18. posted March 18, 2016, https://www.youtube.com/watch?v= FE5JMVI69Ig&feature=emsubs_digest.

2. Edward H. Romond, Edith A. Perez, John Bryant, Vera Suman, Charles E. Geyer, Nancy E. Davidson, Elizabeth Tan-Chiu, Silvana Martino, Soonmyung Paik, Peter A. Kaufman, Sandra M. Swain, Louis Fehrenbacher, Victor Vogel, Daniel W. Visscher, Ann M. Brown, Shaker R. Dakhil, Eleftherios P. Mamounas, Wilma L. Lingle, Pamela M. Klein, and Norman Wolmark, "Trastuzumab Plus Adjuvant Chemotherapy for Operable HER2-Positive Breast Cancer," New England Journal of Medicine 353, no. 16 (2005): 1673–84, doi: 10.1056/NEJMoa052122.

3. World Health Organization, "WHO Model List of Essential Medicines, 19th List," August 2015, http://www.who.int/selection_medicines/committees/expert/20/EML_2015_FINAL_amended_AUG2015.pdf?ua=1.

4. "U.S. Pharmaceutical Sales 2013," Drugs.com, last modified February 2014, http://www.drugs.com/stats/top100/2013/sales. Herceptin is ranked twenty-fourth.

5. "People Living with Cancer Join the Fix the Patent Laws Campaign," Infojustice.org, February 5, 2015, http://infojustice.org/archives/33877.

6. Ibid. See also, "Proposal for the Inclusion of Trastuzumab in the WHO Model List of Essential Medicines for the Treatment of HER2-Positive Breast Cancer," Thiru's Blog, Knowledge Ecology International, January 14, 2013, http://www.who.int/medicines/publications/essentialmedicines/EML2015_8-May-15.pdf.; World Health Organization, "Essential Medicine Selection: 19th Expert Committee Application," last modified May 13, 2016, http://www.who.int/selection_medicines/committees/expert/19/en/.

7. Roche, "Annual Report 2014," http://www.roche.com/gb14e.pdf.

8. World Bank, "World Development Indicators: South Africa," http://data.worldbank.org/country/south-africa#cpwdi (accessed May 13, 2016).

9. "Problematic Patent Laws," REPOST (blog), Infojustice.org, February 3, 2016, http://infojustice.org/archives/35710.

10. Tobeka Daki, telephone interview with the author, March 24, 2016.

11. Fran Quigley, "A Mother Dies Because of Medicine's Cost," Indianapolis Star (November 22, 2016), http://www.indystar.com/story/opinion/2016/11/22/quigley-mother-dies-medicines-cost/94278814/.

12. Quoted in Fix the Patent Laws, "South Africa."

13. Ibid.; "Activists Demand Roche Drops Cost of Vital Breast Cancer Medicine," Fix the Patent Laws, March 31, 2015, http://www.fixthepatentlaws.org/?p=1064.

14. Médecins Sans Frontières/Doctors Without Borders, The Right Shot: Bringing Down Barriers to Affordable and Adapted Vaccines, 2nd ed. (Geneva: MSF Access Campaign, January, 16, 2015), http://www.doctorswithoutborders.org/article/right-shot-bringing-down-barriers-affordable-and-adapted-vaccines-2nd-edition; Justine Boulo, "One in Five African Children Denied Access to Vaccines: Report," Yahoo News, February 24, 2016, http://news.yahoo.com/one-five-african-children-denied-access-vaccines-report-104931158.html; World Health Organization Strategic Advisory Group of Experts on Immunization, 2015 Assessment Report of the Global Vaccine Action Plan, 2015, http://who.int/immunization/global_vaccine_action_plan/SAGE_GVAP_Assessment_Report_2015_BN.pdf.

15. Ramanan Laxminarayan, Precious Matsoso, Suraj Pant, Charles Brower, John-Arne Røttingen, Keith Klugman, and Sally Davies, "Access to Effective Antimicrobials: A Worldwide Challenge," Lancet 387, no. 10014 (2016): 168–75, doi: http://dx.doi.org/10.1016/S0140-6736(15)00474-2.

16. Ibid.

17. Médecins Sans Frontières/Doctors Without Borders, "The Number 1 Killer of Children under the Age of 5," November 10, 2015, http://www.afairshot.org/articles/2015/11/10/the-number-one-killer-of-children-under-5.

18. GAVI, "About GAVI, the Vaccine Alliance," http://www.gavi.org/about/ (accessed May 13, 2016).

19. Médecins Sans Frontières/Doctors Without Borders, "MSF Calls on GSK and Pfizer to Slash Pneumo Vaccine Price to $5 per Child for Poor Countries," January 20, 2015, http://www.msf.org/en/article/access-msf-calls-gsk-and-pfizer-slash-pneumo-vaccine-price-5-child-poor-countries-ahead.

20. Médecins Sans Frontières/Doctors Without Borders, Right Shot, 4.

21. Médecins Sans Frontières/Doctors Without Borders, "MSF Calls."

22. Benedict Cooper, "How the 'Free Market' in Vaccines Is Neither Free nor Fair," New Statesman, March 3, 2016, http://www.newstatesman.com/politics/health/2016/03/how-free-market-vaccines-neither-free-nor-fair. The high price of vaccines means that immunization gaps appear in counterintuitive places: some middle-income countries ineligible for Gavi vaccine support have lower vaccination rates than poorer countries because those middle-income countries are sometimes asked to pay more for vaccines than wealthy nations do. Health

programs in Morocco and Tunisia pay more for the same vaccines than their counterparts in France; Médecins Sans Frontières/Doctors Without Borders, Right Shot, 25.

23. Médecins Sans Frontières/Doctors Without Borders, "MSF Welcomes Pfizer's Pneumonia Vaccine Price Reduction For Children In Humanitarian Emergencies," November 15, 2016, https://www.msf.org.au/article/project-news/msf-welcomes-pfizer%E2%80%99s-pneumonia-vaccine-price-reduction-children-humanitarian.

24. Hans V. Hogerzeil and Zafar Mirza, World Medicines Situation 2011: Access to Essential Medicine as Part of the Right to Health (Geneva: World Health Organization, 2011), 1, http://apps.who.int/medicinedocs/documents/s18772en/s18772en.pdf.

25. United Nations General Assembly, "Promotion and Protection of Human Rights: Human Rights Questions, including Alternative Approaches for Improving the Effective Enjoyment of Human Rights and Fundamental Freedoms," A/63/263, August 11, 2008, http://www.who.int/medicines/areas/human_rights/A63_263.pdf, at 15.

26. World Health Organization, Health in 2015: From MDGs, Millennium Development Goals, to SDGs, Sustainable Development Goals (Washington, DC; World Health Organization, 2015), http://www.who.int/gho/publications/mdgs-sdgs/en/; United Nations Development Programme, "Secretary-General Ban Ki-Moon Issues Call for New Deal on Medicines," news release, December 11, 2015, http://www.undp.org/content/undp/en/home/presscenter/pressreleases/2015/12/11/secretary-general-ban-ki-moon-issues-call-for-new-deal-on-medicines.html.

27. World Health Organization, Health in 2015: From MDGs, Millennium Development Goals, to SDGs, (Sustainable Development Goals), 134. As Dr. Manica Balasegaram, a Médecins Sans Frontières physician, puts it, "Patents create long monopolies, which allow pharmaceutical companies to charge the maximum price they can without fear of competition. Patients and health providers are put in a near-impossible predicament: Either they pay the market rate, or they wait until the maximum profits have been squeezed out of a drug and its patent expires. Waiting in many cases means dying." "Medicine Is Just for Those Who Can Afford It," Al Jazerra, March 14, 2014, http://www.aljazeera.com/indepth/opinion/2014/03/medicine-just-those-who-can-aff-201431181911299288.html.

28. World Health Organization, Health in 2015, 57.

29. Ibid., 107, 118. See, also "The Problem: A Lack of Treatment for Non-Communicable Diseases in Low- and Middle-Income Countries," Young Professionals Chronic Disease Network, https://www.classy.org/events/multiplychange/e58528 (accessed May 17, 2016). Chemotherapy is only available in 32 percent of African countries.

30. World Health Organization, Health in 2015, 57.

31. Ibid., 145.

32. Ibid., 163.

33. Global Commission on Drug Policy, "The Negative Impact of Drug Control on Public Health: The Global Crisis of Avoidable Pain," 2012, http://www.globalcommissionondrugs.org/wp-content/uploads/2012/03/GCODP-THE-NEGATIVE-IMPACT-OF-DRUG-CONTROL-ON-PUBLIC-HEALTH-EN.pdf, 5.

34. Alexandra Cameron, Margaret Ewen, Dennis Ross-Degnan, Douglas Ball, and Richard Laing, "Medicine Prices, Availability, and Affordability in 36 Developing and Middle-Income Countries: A Secondary Analysis," Lancet 373, no. 9659 (2009): 240–49, doi: 10.1016/S0140-6736(08)61762-6.

35. World Health Organization, "WHO Model List of Essential Medicines."

36. Thomas Pogge, "Harnessing the Power of Pharmaceutical Innovation," in The Power of Pills: Social, Ethical, and Legal Issues in Drug Development, Marketing and Pricing, ed. Jillian Claire Cohen, Patricia Illingworth, and Udo Schuklent (London: Pluto Press 2006), 149.

37. United Nations, "Sustainable Development Goals and Targets—Health: Goal 3: Ensure Healthy Lives and Promote Well-Being for All at All Ages," https://sustainabledevelopment.

un.org/sdg3 (accessed November 5, 2016). These targets include 3.8: "Achieve universal health coverage, including . . . access to safe, effective, quality and affordable essential medicines and vaccines for all," and 3.b: "Support the research and development of vaccines and medicines for the communicable and noncommunicable diseases that primarily affect developing countries, provide access to affordable essential medicines and vaccines, in accordance with the Doha Declaration on the TRIPS Agreement and Public Health, which affirms the right of developing countries to use to the full the provisions in the Agreement on Trade Related Aspects of Intellectual Property Rights regarding flexibilities to protect public health, and, in particular, provide access to medicines for all."

38. "Ban Established Eminent Panel to Help Broaden Access to Quality Medicines at Affordable Costs," UN News Centre, November, 20, 2015, http://www.un.org/apps/news/story.asp? NewsID=52614#.VqTb1TbSmM9; UN Secretary General, Report of the United Nations High-Level Panel on Access to Health Technologies, September 2016, https://static1.squarespace.com/static/562094dee4b0d00c1a3ef761/t/57d9c6ebf5e231b2f02c d3d4/1473890031320/UNSG+HLP+Report+FINAL+12+Sept+2016.pdf, 8.

39. Margaret Chan, "Keynote Address to the Regional Committee for the Western Pacific, Sixty-Fifth Session, Manila, Philippines," World Health Organization, October 13, 2014, http://who.int/dg/speeches/2014/regional-committee-western-pacific/en/.

40. Ibid.

41. Charlie Cooper, "Ebola Outbreak: Why Has 'Big Pharma' Failed Deadly Virus' Victims?" Independent, September 6, 2014, http://www.independent.co.uk/life-style/health-and-families/health-news/ebola-outbreak-big-pharma-failed-victims-why-9716615.html.

42. Thomas W Geisbert and Peter B Jahrling, "Towards a Vaccine against Ebola Virus," Expert Review of Vaccines 2 (2003): 89.

43. Cooper, "Ebola Outbreak."

44. "Experts: Ebola Vaccine at Least 50 White People Away," Onion, July 30, 2014, http://www.theonion.com/article/experts-ebola-vaccine-at-least-50-white-people-awa-36580.

45. Chan, "Keynote Address."

4. Cancer Patients Face Particularly Deadly Barriers to Medicines

1. World Health Organization, "Cancer," fact sheet, February 2017, http://www.who.int/mediacentre/factsheets/fs297/en/.

2. Margaret Chan, "WHO Director-General Addresses Ministerial Meeting on Universal Health Coverage," keynote address [transcript], Singapore, Ministerial Meeting on Universal Health Coverage: The Post-2015 Challenge, February 10, 2015, http://www.who.int/dg/speeches/2015/singapore-uhc/en/.

3. Robert Pear, "Medicare, Reversing Itself, Will Pay More for an Expensive New Cancer Drug," New York Times, August 8, 2015, http://www.nytimes.com/2015/08/09/us/medicare-reversing-itself-will-pay-more-for-an-expensive-new-cancer-drug.html?_r=0. In India, Bristol-Meyers Squibb prices a leukemia drug at $108 per day, twenty-five times the average daily income there; Sandeep Kishore, Kavitha Kolappa, Jordan D. Jarvis, Paul H. Park, Rachel Belt, Thirukumaran Balasubramaniam, and Rachel Kiddell-Monroe, "Overcoming Obstacles to Enable Access to Medicines for Noncommunicable Diseases in Poor Countries," Health Affairs 34, no. 9 (2015): 1569–77, doi: 10.1377/hlthaff.2015.0375.

4. IMS Institute for Healthcare Informatics, Developments in Cancer Treatments, Market Dynamics, Patient Access and Value: Global Oncology Trend Report 2015, http://www.imshealth.com/en/thought-leadership/ims-institute/reports/global-oncology-trend-2015.

5. Ibid.; Jonathan D. Rockoff, "How Pfizer Set the Cost of Its New Drug at $9,850 a Month," Wall Street Journal, December 9, 2015, http://www.wsj.com/articles/the-art-of-setting-a-drug-price-1449628081.

6. Hagop Kantarjian, David Steensma, Judit Rius Sanjuan, Adam Elshaug, and Donald Light, "High Cancer Drug Prices in the United States: Reasons and Proposed Solutions, Journal of Oncology Practice, May 6, 2014, http://www.pnhp.org/news/2014/may/high-cancer-drug-prices#.

7. Rockoff, "How Pfizer Set the Cost."

8. "Drug Companies in America: The Costly War on Cancer: New Cancer Drugs Are Technically Impressive. but Must They Cost So Much?" Economist, May 26, 2011, http://www.economist.com/node/18743951.

9. Andrew Hill, Dzintars Gotham, Joseph Fortunak, Jonathan Meldrum, Isabelle Erbacher, Manuel Martin, Haitham Shoman, Jacob Levi, William G. Powderly, and Mark Bower, "Target Prices for Mass Production of Tyrosine Kinase Inhibitors for Global Cancer Treatment," BMJ Open 6, no. 1 (2016), doi: 0.1136/bmjopen-2015-009586.

10. Ibid. Only 5 percent of the global resources for cancer are spent in the developing world, yet those countries account for almost 80 percent of the negative impact of cancer (measured in terms of years lost to illness or death, known as disability adjusted years); "Global Task Force on Expanded Access to Cancer Care and Control: An Initiative Directed by HGEI, HMS, HSPH, FHCRC, UW and UW Med," http://gtfccc.harvard.edu/icb/icb.do?keyword=k69586&tabgroupid=icb.tabgroup138264 (accessed June 5, 2016).

11. "A Cancer Crisis, a Good Solution," Partners in Health, last modified July 1, 2016, http://www.pih.org/blog/a-cancer-crisis-a-good-solution?utm_source=Twitter&utm_medium=Paid+Social&utm_content=RwandaCancerLetter&utm_campaign=Community+Growth+2016.

12. Quoted in James Gallagher, " 'There's No Point Giving Free Cancer Drugs to Africa,' " BBC News, June 9, 2016, http://www.bbc.com/news/health-36482367?SThisFB.

13. Ed Silverman, "Sharp Rise in Cancer Drug Spending Forecast, but Access Remains a Problem," Stat News, June 2, 2016, https://www.statnews.com/pharmalot/2016/06/02/spending-cancer-drugs-forecast-access-still-problem/.

14. Kishore et al., "Overcoming Obstacles."

15. Timothy P. Hanna and Alfred C. T. Kangolle, "Cancer Control in Developing Countries: Using Health Data and Health Services Research to Measure and Improve Access, Quality and Efficiency," Biomed Central International Health and Human Rights 10 (2010), doi: 10.1186/1472-698X-10-24.

16. Ellen t'Hoen, "Access to Cancer Treatment: A Study of Medicine Pricing Issues with Recommendations for Improving Access to Cancer Medication," Oxfam, February 2015, https://www.oxfam.org/sites/www.oxfam.org/files/file_attachments/rr-access-cancer-treatment-inequality-040215-en.pdf, 25; Sarah Boseley, "Big Pharma's Worst Nightmare," Guardian, January 26, 2016, https://www.theguardian.com/society/2016/jan/26/big-pharmas-worst-nightmare.

17. Ayalew Tefferi, Hagop Kantarjian, S. Vincent Rajkumar, Lawrence H. Baker, Jan L. Abkowitz, John W. Adamson, Ranjana Hira Advani, James Allison, Karen H. Antman, Robert C. Bast Jr., John M. Bennett, Edward J. Benz Jr., Nancy Berliner, Joseph Bertino, Ravi Bhatia, Smita Bhatia, Deepa Bhojwani, Charles D. Blanke, Clara D. Bloomfield, Linda Bosserman, Hal E. Broxmeyer, John C. Byrd, Fernando Cabanillas, George Peter Canellos, Bruce A. Chabner, Asher Chanan-Khan, Bruce Cheson, Bayard Clarkson, Susan L. Cohn, Gerardo Colon-Otero, Jorge Cortes, Steven Coutre, Massimo Cristofanilli, Walter J. Curran Jr., George Q. Daley, Daniel J. DeAngelo, H. Joachim Deeg, Lawrence H. Einhorn, Harry P. Erba, Francisco J. Esteva, Elihu Estey, Isaiah J. Fidler, James Foran, Stephen Forman, Emil Freireich, Charles Fuchs, James N. George, Morie A. Gertz, Sergio Giralt, Harvey Golomb, Peter Greenberg, Jordan Gutterman, Robert I. Handin, Samuel Hellman, Paulo Marcelo

Hoff, Ronald Hoffman, Waun Ki Hong, Mary Horowitz, Gabriel N. Hortobagyi, Clifford Hudis, Jean Pierre Issa, Bruce Evan Johnson, Philip W. Kantoff, Kenneth Kaushansky, David Khayat, Fadlo R. Khuri, Thomas J. Kipps, Margaret Kripke, Robert A. Kyle, Richard A. Larson, Theodore S. Lawrence, Ross Levine, Michael P. Link, Scott M. Lippman, Sagar Lonial, Gary H. Lyman, Maurie Markman, John Mendelsohn, Neal J. Meropol, Yoav Messinger, Therese M. Mulvey, Susan O'Brien, Roman Perez-Soler, Raphael Pollock, Josef Prchal, Oliver Press, Jerald Radich, Kanti Rai, Saul A. Rosenberg, Jacob M. Rowe, Hope Rugo, Carolyn D. Runowicz, Brenda M. Sandmaier, Alan Saven, Andrew I. Schafer, Charles Schiffer, Mikkael A. Sekeres, Richard T. Silver, Lillian L. Siu, David P. Steensma, F. Marc Stewart, Wendy Stock, Richard Stone, Rainer Storb, Louise C. Strong, Martin S. Tallman, Michael Thompson, Naoto T. Ueno, Richard A. Van Etten, Julie M. Vose, Peter H. Wiernik, Eric P. Winer, Anas Younes, Andrew D. Zelenetz, and Charles A. LeMaistre, "In Support of a Patient-Driven Initiative and Petition to Lower the High Cost of Cancer Drugs," Mayo Clinic Proceedings 90, no. 8 (2015): 996–1000, http://www.mayoclinicproceedings.org/article/S0025-6196(15)00430-9/pdf.

18. Brian Bolwell, "Many Cancer Patients Must Face Bankruptcy—Or Die," Newsweek, August 13, 2016, http://www.newsweek.com/many-cancer-patients-must-face-bankrupty-or-die-489596.

19. "How Einhorn Helped Turn a Deadly Cancer into a Curable Disease," OncLive, May 28, 2014, http://www.onclive.com/publications/oncology-live/2014/may-2014/how-einhorn-helped-turn-a-deadly-cancer-into-a-curable-disease.

20. Ibid.

21. Ibid.

22. Quoted in Fran Quigley, "Push Drugmakers to Lower Price of Cancer Medicine," Indianapolis Star, August 18, 2015, http://www.indystar.com/story/opinion/2015/08/18/quigley-push-drugmakers-lower-price-cancer-medicine/31905253/.

23. Jeanne Whalen, "Doctors Object to High Cancer-Drug Prices," Wall Street Journal, July 23, 2015, http://www.wsj.com/articles/doctors-object-to-high-cancer-drug-prices-1437 624060.

24. Experts in Chronic Myeloid Leukemia, "The Price of Drugs for Chronic Myeloid Leukemia (CML) Is a Reflection of the Unsustainable Prices of Cancer Drugs: From the Perspective of a Large Group of CML Experts," Blood 121, no. 22 (2013): 4439–42, doi: 10.1182/blood-2013-03-49000.

25. Peter B. Bach, Leonard B. Saltz, and Robert Wittes, "In Cancer Care, Cost Matters," New York Times, October 15, 2012, http://www.nytimes.com/2012/10/15/opinion/a-hospital-says-no-to-an-11000-a-month-cancer-drug.html?_r=0.

26. Quoted in Gardiner Harris, "Waste in Cancer Drugs Costs $3 Billion a Year, a Study Says," New York Times, March 1, 2016, http://www.nytimes.com/2016/03/01/health/waste-in-cancer-drugs-costs-3-billion-a-year-a-study-says.html?_r=0'ch. See also Peter Bach, Rena Conti, Raymond Muller, Geoffrey Schnorr, and Leonard Saltz, "Yes, Providing Cancer Drugs in Multiple Vial Sizes Could Save Patients and Taxpayers Money," Health Affairs Blog, June 8, 2016, http://healthaffairs.org/blog/2016/06/08/yes-providing-cancer-drugs-in-multiple-vial-sizes-could-save-patients-and-payers-money/.

27. Public Citizen, "Patient Groups and Big Pharma," news release, August 4, 2016, http://www.citizen.org/patients-groups-and-big-pharma-funding-report.

28. Katie Thomas, "Furor over Drug Prices Puts Patient Advocacy Groups in Bind," New York Times, September 27, 2016, http://www.nytimes.com/2016/09/28/business/furor-over-drug-prices-puts-patient-advocacy-groups-in-bind.html?_r=0.

29. Public Citizen, "Patient Groups and Big Pharma"; David S. Hilzenrath, "In FDA Meetings, 'Voice' of the Patient Often Funded by Drug Companies," Project on Government

Oversight, December 1, 2016, http://www.pogo.org/our-work/reports/2016/in-fda-meetings-voice-of-the-patient-often-funded-by-drug-companies.html.

30. Institute for Health and Socio-Economic Policy, Health Advocates or Hired Guns?: Critics of Prop 61 Receive Millions from the Pharmaceutical Industry (Orinda, CA: Institute for Health and Socio-Economic Policy, 2016), http://nurses.3cdn.net/76f4ad8ec2b366d306_zum6btegn.pdf.

31. Jennifer Hinkel, comment on Trudy Lieberman, "Groups Push Pharma Agenda under the Guise of Patient Advocacy," HealthNewsReview, February 10, 2016 (posted 10:22 p.m.), http://www.healthnewsreview.org/2016/02/groups-push-pharma-agenda-under-the-guise-of-patient-advocacy/.

32. Barbara Mintzes, "Should Patient Groups Accept Money from Drug Companies? No," BMJ 334, no. 7600 (2007): 935, doi: 10.1136/bmj.39185.394005.AD.

33. Quoted in Fran Quigley, "A Bitter Pill: Can the Access to Medicines Movement Score Another Victory?" Foreign Affairs, October 8, 2015, https://www.foreignaffairs.com/articles/south-africa/2015-10-18/bitter-pill.

5. The Current Medicine System Neglects Many Major Diseases

1. Adam Mannan and Alan Story, "Abolishing the Product Patent: A Step Forward for Global Access to Drugs," in Power of Pills: Social, Ethical and Legal Issues in Drug Development, Marketing and Pricing, ed. Jillian Clare Cohen, Patricia Illingworth and Udo Schüklenk (Ann Arbor, MI: Pluto Press, 2006), 183.

2. Ibid.

3. Global Network for Neglected Tropical Diseases, "About: Our Mission," last modified 2015, http://www.globalnetwork.org/about.

4. Belen Pedrique, Nathalie Strub-Wourgaft, Claudette Some, Piero Olliaro, Patrice Trouiller, Nathan Ford, Bernard Pécoul, and Jean-Hervé Bradol, "The Drug and Vaccine Landscape for Neglected Diseases (2000–11): A Systematic Assessment," Lancet 1, no. 6 (2013): e371–e379, doi: http://dx.doi.org/10.1016/S2214-109X(13)70078-0.

5. John-Arne Røttingen, Sadie Regmi, Mari Eide, Alison J. Young, Roderik F. Viergever, Christine Årdal, Javier Guzman, Danny Edwards, Stephen A. Matlin, and Robert F. Terry, "Mapping of Available Health Research and Development Data: What's There, What's Missing, and What Role Is There for a Global Observatory?" Lancet 382, no. 990 (2013):1286–307, doi: http://dx.doi.org/10.1016/S0140-6736(13)61046-6.

6. Pierre Chirac and Els Torreele, "Global Framework on Essential Health R&D," Lancet 382, no. 9522 (2006):1560–61, doi: http://dx.doi.org/10.1016/S0140-6736(06)68672-8.

7. Sheila Davey, ed., The 10/90 Report on Health Research 2000 (Geneva: Global Forum for Health Research, World Health Organization, 2000), http://announcementsfiles.cohred.org/gfhr_pub/assoc/s14791e/s14791e.pdf.

8. World Health Organization, Global Tuberculosis Report 2015, 20th ed., http://www.who.int/tb/publications/global_report/gtbr2015_executive_summary.pdf?ua=1.

9. Jane Andrews, "To Be or Not to Be Exclusive: The Sutezolid Story," Lancet 4, no. 2 (2016): e89–e90, doi: http://dx.doi.org/10.1016/S2214-109X(15)00285-5. One little-referenced casualty of the neglect of research on impactful diseases is the disappointment of biomedical researchers who had hoped to devote their life work to developing new lifesaving medicines instead of copycat drugs and drugs that address the perceived lifestyle needs of the global wealthy; Sebastian Krueger and Els Torreele, "Torching the Myths of Expensive Medicines," Open Society Foundations, September 10, 2013, https://www.opensocietyfoundations.org/voices/torching-myths-expensive-medicines.

10. Andrews, "To Be or Not"; Mark Harrington, letter to Carol Nancy, Chairman of the Board and Chief Executive Officer Sequella Inc., July 22, 2013, http://www.tbonline.info/media/uploads/documents/letter_to_sequella_re_sutezolid.pdf.

11. Treatment Action Group, 2013 Report on Tuberculosis Research Funding Trends, 2005–2012, http://www.treatmentactiongroup.org/sites/g/files/g450272/f/201310/TAG_TB_2013_8.5_slides.r5.pdf.

12. Shilpa Phadnis, "Astra Zeneca to Shut Avishkar R&D Site in Bangalore," Times of India, January 31, 2014, http://timesofindia.indiatimes.com/business/india-business/Astra Zeneca-to-shut-Avishkar-RD-site-in-Bangalore/articleshow/29669606.cms.

13. Fatima Hansia, "Big Pharma Abandons New Tuberculosis Drug Research," Corp-Watch (blog), April 1, 2014, http://www.corpwatch.org/article.php?id=15939.

14. Andrew Ward, "Download Big Pharma Balks at Investment in TB," Financial Times, March 24, 2014, http://www.ft.com/intl/cms/s/0/417dee98-a52a-11e3-8988-00144feab7de. html#axzz43MGQmGyL.

15. Kai Kupferschmidt, "Long-Awaited Report Outlines How to Fight Antimicrobial Resistance—And How To Pay For It," Science, May 18, 2016, http://www.sciencemag.org/news/2016/05/long-awaited-report-outlines-how-fight-antimicrobial-resistance-and-how-pay-it.

16. Veronika J. Wirtz, Hans V. Hogerzeil, Andrew L. Gray, Maryam Bigdeli, Corne-lis P. de Joncheere, Margaret A. Ewen, Martha Gyansa-Lutterodt, Sun Jing, Vera L. Luiza, Regina M Mbindyo, Helene Möller, Corrina Moucheraud, Bernard Pécoul, Lembit Rägo, Arash Rashidian, Dennis Ross-Degnan, Peter N. Stephens, Yot Teerawattananon, Ellen F. M. 't Hoen, Anita K. Wagner, Prashant Yadav, Michael R. Reich, "Essential Medicines for Universal Health Coverage," The Lancet, November 7, 2016, http://yolse.org/wp-content/uploads/2016/11/EssentialMeds.pdf, 57.

17. Andrew Jack, "Novartis Chief in Warning on Cheap Drugs," Financial Times, September 30, 2006, http://www.ft.com/cms/s/0/6cfd37e8-5020-11db-9d85-0000779e2340.html.

18. Els Torreele, "Only a Radical Overhaul Can Reclaim Medicines for the Public Interest," PLoS (blog), October 13, 2015, http://blogs.plos.org/yoursay/2015/10/13/talking-about-drug-prices-access-to-medicines/.

19. Donald Light and Rebecca Warburton, "Demythologizing the High Costs of Pharmaceutical Research," BioSocieties 6, no. 1 (2011): 34–50, quotation on 47, doi: 10.1057/biosoc.2010.40; Deena Beasley, "U.S. Regulator Says Too Many Drugmakers Chasing Same Cancer Strategy," Reuters, June 14, 2016, http://mobile.reuters.com/article/idUSKCN0YW15 T?feedType=RSS&feedName=healthNews&utm_source=feedburner&utm_medium=feed&utm_campaign=Feed%253A+reuters%252FhealthNews+%2528Reuters+Health+News%2529.

20. Joshua J. Gagne and Niteesh Choudhry, "How Many "Me-Too" Drugs Is Too Many?" Journal of the American Medical Association 305, no. 7 (2011): 711–712, doi: 10.1001/jama.2011.152. Unfortunately, there is virtually no price competition in the "me-too" market; Aidan Hollis, "Me-Too Drugs: Is There a Problem," University of Calgary, Calgary, Canada, December 13, 2004, http://www.who.int/intellectualproperty/topics/ip/Me-tooDrugs_Hollis1.pdf.

21. Marcia Angell, The Truth about the Drug Companies: How They Deceive Us and What to Do about It (New York: Random House, 2005), 76–81, 86.

22. Claire Cassedy, "Transcript of Bayer CEO Marjin Dekkers Quote at the December 3, 2013 FT Event, Regarding India Compulsory License of Nexavar," Knowledge Ecology International, Claire Cassedy's Blog, February 7, 2014, http://keionline.org/node/1924.

6. Corporate Research and Development Investments Are Exaggerated

1. Quoted in Marcia Angell, The Truth about the Drug Companies: How They Deceive Us and What to Do about It (New York: Random House, 2005), 38.

2. Tufts Center for the Study of Drug Development, "Cost to Develop and Win Marketing Approval for a New Drug Is $2.6 Billion," November 18, 2014, http://csdd.tufts.edu/news/complete_story/pr_tufts_csdd_2014_cost_study.

3. John J. Castellani, "Contrasting Perspectives on the Price of Medicine," New York Times, January 26, 2015, http://www.nytimes.com/2015/01/26/opinion/contrasting-perspectives-on-the-price-of-medicines.html?_r=0; PhRMA, Biopharmaceutical Research & Development: The Process behind New Medicines, August 20, 2015, 1 http://www.phrma.org/sites/default/files/pdf/rd_brochure_022307.pdf.

4. Tufts Center for the Study of Drug Development, "Financial Disclosure," http://csdd.tufts.edu/about/financial_disclosure (accessed June 9, 2016).

5. Joseph A. Di Masi, letter to Manon Ress, Union for Affordable Cancer Treatment, Tufts Center for the Study of Drug Development, March 2, 2015, http://csdd.tufts.edu/files/uploads/DiMasi_Response_to_UACT.pdf; Intellectual Property Watch, "Inside Views: Questions about Funding, Text of Tufts Study on Drug Costs," March 2, 2015, http://www.ip-watch.org/2015/02/03/questions-about-funding-text-of-tufts-study-on-drug-costs/; Aaron E. Carroll, "$2.6 Billion to Develop a Drug? New Estimate Makes Questionable Assumptions," New York Times, November 18, 2014, http://www.nytimes.com/2014/11/19/upshot/calculating-the-real-costs-of-developing-a-new-drug.html?emc=eta1&_r=0.

6. Donald Light and Rebecca Warburton, "Demythologizing the High Costs of Pharmaceutical Research," BioSocieties 6, no. 1 (2011): 34–50, doi: 10.1057/biosoc.2010.40.

7. Ibid., 38, 41. Jerry Avorn, "The $2.6 Billion Pill: Methodologic and Policy Considerations," New England Journal of Medicine 372 (2015): 1877–79.

8. Ibid., 39.

9. Ibid.

10. Ibid., 42.

11. Ibid., 42–43.

12. Quoted in Ben Hirschler, "GlaxoSmithKline Boss Says New Drugs Can Be Cheaper," Reuters, March 14, 2013, http://www.reuters.com/article/us-glaxosmithkline-prices-idUSBRE92D0RM20130314.

13. "Billion Dollar Babies: The High Cost of R&D Is Used to Explain Why Drugs Giants Merge, and Why They Must Charge High Prices. The Reality Is Somewhat Different," Economist, November, 28, 2015, http://www.economist.com/news/business/21679203-high-cost-rd-used-explain-why-drugs-giants-merge-and-why-they-must-charge.

14. Universities Allied for Essential Medicines, "Make Medicines for People, Not Profit," last mod. Nov. 2015, https://uaem.wufoo.com/forms/make-medicines-for-people-not-for-profit/.

15. PhRMA, Biopharmaceutical Research & Development, 1; Light and Warburton, "Demythologizing," 43.

16. Light and Warburton, "Demythologizing," 48.

17. Drugs for Neglected Diseases Initiative, "An Innovative Approach to R&D for Neglected Patients. Ten Years of Experience and Lessons Learned by DNDi," news release, January 2014, http://www.dndi.org/?s=+Ten+years+of+experience+and+lessons+learned+by+DNDi.

18. Global Alliance for Tuberculosis Drug Development, Executive Summary for the Economics of TB Drug Development, October 2001, 3, http://www.tballiance.org/downloads/publications/TBA_Economics_Report_Exec.pdf.

19. PhRMA, Vaccine Factbook 2013, 2013, http://www.phrma.org/sites/default/files/pdf/PhRMA_Vaccine_FactBook_2013.pdf; Donald Light, John Kim Andrus, and Rebecca Nunn

Warburton, "Estimated Research and Development Costs of Rotavirus Vaccines," Vaccine 27, no. 47 (2009) 47: 6627–33, doi: 10.1016/j.vaccine.2009.07.077. Francis E. André. "How the Research-Based Industry Approaches Vaccine Development and Establishes Priorities," Developments in Biologicals 110 (2001): 25–29.

20. Meredith Cohn, "Industry Funds Six Times More Clinical Trials Than Feds, Research Shows," Baltimore Sun, December 15, 2015, http://www.baltimoresun.com/health/bs-hs-trial-funding-20151214-story.html.

21. Carolyn Y. Johnson, "This Drug Is Defying a Rare Form of Leukemia—and It Keeps Getting Pricier," Washington Post, March 9, 2016, https://www.washingtonpost.com/business/this-drug-is-defying-a-rare-form-of-leukemia—and-it-keeps-getting-pricier/2016/03/09/4fff8102-c571-11e5-a4aa-f25866ba0dc6_story.html.

22. James Love, "R& D Costs for Gleevec," James Love's Blog, Knowledge Ecology International, April 2, 2013, http://keionline.org/node/1697. Another analysis of drug research and development costs, this time the Bayer research investment into sorafenib, put the estimated cost at $295.7 million, 11 percent of the $2.5 billion Bayer claimed to have invested; James Love, "IPAB Hearing on the Nexavar Compulsory License, Part 1, R&D Costs," James Love's Blog, Knowledge Ecology International, January 19, 2013, http://keionline.org/node/1640.

23. Alfred Engelberg, "How Government Policy Promotes High Drug Prices," Health Affairs (blog), October 29, 2015, http://healthaffairs.org/blog/2015/10/29/how-government-policy-promotes-high-drug-prices/; James Love, "Pharmaceutical Global R&D Was 7.9 Percent of Sales in 2010," James Love's Blog, Knowledge Ecology International, June 9, 2011, http://keionline.org/node/1152.

24. James Love, "Drug Pricing Is Out of Control, What Should be Done?" PLoS (blog), October 19, 2015, http://blogs.plos.org/yoursay/2015/10/19/talking-drug-prices-pt-4-drug-pricing-is-out-of-control-what-should-be-done-by-james-love/.

25. PhRMA, Biopharmaceutical Research & Development.

26. Arlene Weintraub, "Potential for Deals Drives a Big Surge in Biotech Sector," New York Times, July 11, 2013, http://dealbook.nytimes.com/2013/07/11/biotech-companies-surge-as-investors-flock-to-them/?_r=0.

27. Nils Behnke Michael Retterath, Todd Sangster, and Ashish Singh, "New Paths to Value Creation for Pharma," Bain Brief, Bain & Company, September 24, 2014, http://www.bain.com/Images/BAIN_BRIEF_New_paths_to_value_creation_in_pharma.pdf, 3; "Billion Dollar Babies."

28. Quoted in Eric Bender, "Q&A: Bernard Munos," Nature 533, Suppl. 59 (2016), doi: 10.1038/533S59a.

29. Ed Silverman, "Regeneron CEO Spars with Counterparts, Calling Many Price Hikes 'Ridiculous,'" STAT, December 2, 2016, https://www.statnews.com/pharmalot/2016/12/02/regeneron-drug-prices-pfizer/.

30. Lewis Krauskopf and Anand Basu, "Gilead Bets $11 Billion on Hepatitis in Pharmasset Deal," Reuters, November 21, 2011, http://www.reuters.com/article/us-gilead-pharmasset-idUSTRE7AK0XU20111121.

31. Gautam Naik, "GlaxoSmithKline Actively Pursues Drug Licenses," Wall Street Journal, February 13, 2002.

7. The Current System Wastes Billions on Drug Marketing

1. GlobalData, "Top 30 Pharma Companies Spent $112 Billion on Research and Development in 2013, Says GlobalData," news release, December 17, 2014, https://healthcare.globaldata.com/media-center/press-releases/pharmaceuticals/top-30-pharma-companies-spent-112-billion-on-research-and-development-in-2013-says-globaldata; Richard Anderson,

"Pharmaceutical Industry Gets High on Fat Profits," BBC News, November 6, 2014, http://www.bbc.com/news/business-28212223; "Is There a Cure for High Drug Prices?" Consumer Reports, July 29, 2016, http://www.consumerreports.org/drugs/cure-for-high-drug-prices/.

2. Anderson, "Pharmaceutical Industry."

3. "Pfizer Hikes Prices for over 100 Drugs on January 1," Reuters, January 8, 2016, http://www.nbcnews.com/business/business-news/pfizer-hikes-prices-over-100-drugs-january-1-n493281.

4. World Health Organization, "Direct-to-Consumer Advertising under Fire," Bulletin of the World Health Organization 87, no. 8 (2009): 565–644, http://www.who.int/bulletin/volumes/87/8/09-040809/en/.

5. American Medical Association, "AMA Calls for Ban on Direct to Consumer Advertising of Prescription Drugs and Medical Devices," news release, November 17, 2015, http://www.ama-assn.org/ama/pub/news/news/2015/2015-11-17-ban-consumer-prescription-drug-advertising.page; Rebecca Robbins, "Drug Makers Now Spend $5 Billion a Year on Advertising," STAT, March 9, 2016, https://www.statnews.com/2016/03/09/drug-industry-advertising/.

6. Robert A. Bell, Richard L. Kravitz, and Michael S. Wilkes, "Direct-to-Consumer Prescription Drug Advertising and the Public," Journal of General Internal Medicine 14, no. 11 (1999): 651–57, doi: 10.1046/j.1525-1497.1999.01049.x.

7. Mark Peyrot, Neil M. Alperstein, Doris Van Doren, and Laurence G. Poli, "Direct-to-Consumer Ads Can Influence Behavior; Advertising Increases Consumer Knowledge and Prescription Drug Requests," Marketing Health Services 18, no. 2 (1998): 26–32, http://www.ncbi.nlm.nih.gov/pubmed/10180332.

8. Richard L. Kravitz, Ronald M. Epstein, Mitchell D. Feldman, Carol E. Franz, Rahman Azari, Michael S. Wilkes, Ladson Hinton, and Peter Franks, "Influence of Patients' Requests for Direct-to-Consumer Advertised Antidepressants: A Randomized Controlled Trial," Journal of the American Medical Association 293, no. 16 (2005): 1995–2002, doi: 10.1001/jama.293.16.1995.

9. Alfred Engelberg, "How Government Policy Promotes High Drug Prices," Health Affairs (blog), October 29, 2015, http://healthaffairs.org/blog/2015/10/29/how-government-policy-promotes-high-drug-prices/.

10. American Medical Association, "AMA Calls for Ban."

11. "STAT's Stats of the Year: 2016 in Numbers," STAT, December 28, 2016, https://www.statnews.com/2016/12/28/stat-stats-year-in-numbers/; Robbins, "Drug Makers"; Rebecca Robbins, "Get Ready for More Drug Ads: Facebook Is Making a Bid for Pharma Dollars," STAT, November 1, 2016, https://www.statnews.com/2016/11/01/facebook-pharma-drug-ads/.

12. Pew Charitable Trusts, "Fact Sheet: Persuading the Prescribers: Pharmaceutical Industry Marketing and Its Influence on Physicians and Patients," last modified November 11, 2013, http://www.pewtrusts.org/en/research-and-analysis/fact-sheets/2013/11/11/persuading-the-prescribers-pharmaceutical-industry-marketing-and-its-influence-on-physicians-and-patients.

13. Eric G. Campbell, "Doctors and Drug Companies—Scrutinizing Influential Relationships," New England Journal of Medicine 357 (2007): 1796–97, doi: 10.1056/NEJMp078141.

14. Pew Charitable Trusts, "Fact Sheet: Persuading the Prescribers."

15. Joseph Engelberg, Christopher A. Parsons, and Nathan Tefft, "Financial Conflicts of Interest in Medicine," Rady School of Management, University of South California, San Diego, January 2014, http://rady.ucsd.edu/faculty/directory/engelberg/pub/portfolios/DOCTORS.pdf.

16. Jared S. Hopkins, "Doctors Getting Free Meals Pick Branded Drugs More, Study Finds," Bloomberg News, June 20, 2016, http://www.bloomberg.com/news/articles/2016-

06-20/doctors-getting-free-meals-pick-branded-drugs-more-study-finds. See also Ryann Gro-chowski Jones and Charles Ornstein, "Matching Industry Payments to Medicare Prescrib-ing Patterns: An Analysis," ProPublica, March 2016, https://static.propublica.org/projects/d4d/20160317-matching-industry-payments.pdf?22.

17. Kenneth Katz, Erika E. Reid, and Mary-Margaret Chren, "Drug Samples in Derma-tology: Out of the Closet, into the Dustbin," Journal of the American Medical Association: Dermatology 150, no. 5 (2014): 483–85, doi: 10.1001/jamadermatol.2013.9711. See also Robert Cialdini, Influence: The Psychology of Persuasion (HarperCollins, 2007), 27: "The beauty of the free sample . . . is that it is also a gift and, as such, can engage the reciprocity rule."

18. Ed Silverman, "What Generics? Americans Spend an Extra $73b for Name-Brand Meds," STAT, May 9, 2016, https://www.statnews.com/pharmalot/2016/05/09/generics-drug-prices-cholesterol/.

8. The Current System Compromises Physician Integrity and Leads to Unethical Corporate Behavior

1. Pew Charitable Trusts, "Fact Sheet: Persuading the Prescribers: Pharmaceutical Indus-try Marketing and Its Influence on Physicians and Patients," last modified November 11, 2013, http://www.pewtrusts.org/en/research-and-analysis/fact-sheets/2013/11/11/persuading-the-prescribers-pharmaceutical-industry-marketing-and-its-influence-on-physicians-and-patients.

2. Eric G. Campbell, Joel S. Weissman, Susan Ehringhaus, Sowmya R. Rao, Beverly Moy, Sandra Feibelmann, and Susan Dorr Goold, "Institutional Academic-Industry Rela-tionships," Journal of the American Medical Association 298, no. 15 (2007): 1779–86, doi: 10.1001/jama.298.15.1779.

3. Matt Lamkin and Carl Elliott, "Curing the Disobedient Patient: Medication Adher-ence Programs as Pharmaceutical Marketing Tools," Journal of Medical Ethics 42, no. 4 (2014): 492–500, doi: 10.1111/jlme.12170.

4. Alfred Engelberg, "How Government Policy Promotes High Drug Prices," Health Affairs, October 29, 2015, http://healthaffairs.org/blog/2015/10/29/how-government-policy-promotes-high-drug-prices/.

5. Bianca DiJulio, Jamie Firth, and Mollyann Brodie, Kaiser Health Tracking Poll: August 2015 (Menlo Park, CA: Kaiser Family Foundation, 2015), http://kff.org/health-costs/poll-finding/kaiser-health-tracking-poll-august-2015/. See also Gallup, "Business and Indus-try Sector Ratings," August 3–7, 2016, http://www.gallup.com/poll/12748/business-indus-try-sector-ratings.aspx. The pharmaceutical industry is ranked as the least respected private industry.

6. Ben Goldacre, Bad Pharma: How Drug Companies Mislead Doctors and Harm Patients (London: Faber and Faber, 2012), xv.

7. Jason Dana and George Loewenstein, "A Social Science Perspective on Gifts to Phy-sicians from Industry," Journal of the American Medical Association 290, no. 2 (2003): 252–55, doi: 10.1001/jama.290.2.252; Sunita Sah and Adriane Fugh-Berman, "Physicians under the Influence: Social Psychology and Industry Marketing Strategies," Journal of Law and Medical Ethics 41, no. 3 (2013): 665–72, doi: 10.1111/jlme.12076.

8. Catherine D. DeAngelis and Phil B. Fontanarosa, "Impugning the Integrity of Medical Science: The Adverse Effects of Industry Influence," Journal of the American Medical Associ-ation 299, no. 15 (2008): 1833–35, doi: 10.1001/jama.299.15.1833.

9. American Medical Association, "Physician Financial Transparency Reports (Sunshine Act)," 1995–2016, http://www.ama-assn.org/ama/pub/advocacy/topics/sunshine-act-and-physi cian-financial-transparency-reports.page (accessed June 12, 2016).

10. Campbell et al., "Institutional Academic-Industry Relationships."

11. Daniel Wikkler, "A Crisis in the Medical Profession: Time for Flexner II," in Ethics and the Business of Biomedicine, ed. Denis G. Arnold (Cambridge, UK: Cambridge University Press, 2009), 251. Concern over the impact of pharmaceutical corporate payments on experts' objectivity goes beyond the academic medicine community; Eric Lipton, Nicholas Confessore, and Brooke Williams, "Think Tank Scholar or Corporate Consultant? It Depends on the Day," New York Times, August 8, 2016, http://www.nytimes.com/2016/08/09/us/pol itics/think-tank-scholars-corporate-consultants.html.

12. Adriane Fugh-Berman, "How Basic Scientists Help the Pharmaceutical Industry Market Drugs," PLoS Biology 11, no. 11 (2013): e1001716, doi: 10.1371/journal.pbio.1001716.

13. Ibid.

14. Quoted in Wikkler, "Crisis in the Medical Profession," 251.

15. Ibid. 250–51.

16. Andreas Lundh, Sergio Sismondo, Joel Lexchin, Octavian A Busuioc, and Lisa Bero, "Industry Sponsorship and Research Outcome," Cochrane Database of Systematic Reviews 12 (2012), doi: 10.1002/14651858.MR000033.pub2; Konstantinos K. Tsilidis, Orestis A. Panagiotou, Emily S. Sena, Eleni Aretouli, Evangelos Evangelou, David W. Howells, Rustam Al-Shahi Salman, Malcolm R. Macleod, and John P. A. Ioannidis, "Evaluation of Excess Significance Bias in Animal Studies of Neurological Diseases," PLoS Biology 11, no. 7 (2013): e1001609, doi: 10.1371/journal.pbio.1001609; Tongeji Tungaraza and Rob Poole, "Influence of Drug Company Authorship and Sponsorship on Drug Trial Outcomes, British Journal of Psychiatry 191, no. 1 (2007): 82–83, doi: 10.1192/bjp.bp.106.024547.

17. Fugh-Berman, "How Basic Scientists."

18. Ibid.

19. Ed Silverman, "Increase in Industry-Funded Drug Trials Bad for Public Health, Researcher Says," STAT, December 16, 2015, http://www.statnews.com/pharmalot/2015/12/16/ pharmalot-nih-drug-trials/.

20. Goldacre, Bad Pharma 341.

21. Marcia Angell, The Truth about the Drug Companies: How They Deceive Us and What to Do about It (New York: Random House, 2005).

22. Thomy Tonia, Guido Schwarzer, and Julia Bohlius, "Cancer, Meta-Analysis and Reporting Biases: The Case of Erythropoiesis-Stimulating Agents," Swiss Medical Weekly, May 7, 2013, doi:10.4414/smw.2013.13776; Charles L. Bennett, "Association between Pharmaceutical Support and Basic Science Research on Erythropoiesis-Stimulating Agents," Archives of Internal Medicine 170, no. 16 (2010): 1490–98, doi: 10.1001/archinternmed.2010.309.

23. Joseph Ross, Kevin P. Hill, David Egilman, and Harlan M. Krumholz, "Guest Authorship and Ghostwriting in Publications Related to Rofecoxib: A Case Study of Industry Documents from Rofecoxib Litigation," Journal of the American Medical Association 299, no. 15 (2008): 1800–1817, doi: 10.1001/jama.299.15.1800; Bruce Psaty and Richard Kronmal, "Reporting Mortality Findings in Trials of Rofecoxib for Alzheimer Disease or Cognitive Impairment: A Case Study Based on Documents from Rofecoxib Litigation," Journal of the American Medical Association 299, no. 15 (2008): 1813–17, doi: 10.1001/ jama.299.15.1813.

24. Fugh-Berman, "How Basic Scientists."

25. Jerome P. Kassirer, On the Take: How Medicine's Complicity with Big Business Can Endanger Your Health (New York: Oxford University Press, 2005); John Abramson,

Overdosed America: The Broken Promise of American Medicine (New York: Harper Perennial, 2004); Jerry Avorn, Powerful Medicines: The Benefits, Costs and Risks of Prescription Drugs (New York: Vintage Books, 2004); Angell, The Truth about the Drug Companies.

26. Marcia Angell, "Is Academic Medicine for Sale?" New England Journal of Medicine 342 (2000): 1516–18, doi: 10.1056/NEJM200005183422009.

27. Thomas J. Ruane, "Letter to Editor," New England Journal of Medicine 343 (2000): 510, doi: 1056/NEJM200008173430712.

28. Quoted in Sarah Lueck, "Drug Prices Far Outpace Inflation: Report by Consumer Group Highlights Cost Pressures Faced by Senior Citizens," Wall Street Journal, July 10, 2003, http://www.wsj.com/articles/SB105779249051280400.

29. Quoted in Rufus Pollock, "Strong Words from WHO on Pharma Industry," blog, May 29, 2016, http://rufuspollock.org/2016/05/29/strong-words-from-who-on-pharma-industry/.

30. Transparency International UK, "Corruption in the Pharmaceutical Sector: Diagnosing the Challenges," June 2016, 5, http://www.transparency.org.uk/publications/corruption-in-the-pharmaceutical-sector/.

31. Sammy Almashat, Charles Preston, Timothy Waterman, Sidney Wolfe, and the Public Citizen's Health Research Group, Rapidly Increasing Criminal and Civil Penalties against the Pharmaceutical Industry: 1991 to 2001 (Washington, DC: Public Citizen's Health Research Group, December 16, 2010), 5, http://www.citizen.org/hrg1924.

32. Ibid., 5–6.

33. Ibid., 10, 19.

34. Ibid., 9.

35. Ibid., 15.

36. James O'Toole, "Pfizer Settles Foreign Bribery Charges," CNN Money, August 7, 2012, http://money.cnn.com/2012/08/07/news/companies/pfizer-bribery-charges/index.htm; Seth Stern, "GlaxoSmithKline Agrees to Pay $3 Billion in U.S. Drug Settlement," Bloomberg Business, July 7, 2012, http://www.bloomberg.com/news/articles/2012-07-02/glaxosmithkline-agrees-to-pay-3-billion-in-u-s-drug-settlement.

37. Public Citizen, "Pharmaceutical Industry Is Biggest Defrauder of the Federal Government under the False Claims Act," December 10, 2010, http://www.citizen.org/Page.aspx?pid=4734#table; Almashat et al., Rapidly Increasing Criminal and Civil Penalties, 15.

38. Federal Trade Commission, "Bristol-Meyers-Squibb Company," last modified March 31, 2009, https://www.ftc.gov/enforcement/cases-proceedings/0610235/bristol-myers-squibb-company.

39. Harriet Ryan, Lisa Girion, and Scott Glover, " 'You Want a Description of Hell?' Oxycontin's 12-Hour Problem," Los Angeles Times, May 5, 2016, http://www.latimes.com/projects/oxycontin-part1/. Sandra Tan, "Other Counties Expected to Follow Erie County In Suing Makers Of Narcotic Painkillers," Buffalo News, February 3, 2017, http://buffalonews.com/2017/02/03/counties-expected-follow-erie-county-suing-makers-narcotic-pain-killers/.

40. Christopher Ingraham, "One Striking Chart Shows Why Pharma Companies Are Fighting Legal Marijuana," Washington Post, July 13, 2016, https://www.washingtonpost.com/news/wonk/wp/2016/07/13/one-striking-chart-shows-why-pharma-companies-are-fighting-legal-marijuana/?utm_term=.4ef20d0ee35f.

41. Andrew Ward and Ralph Atkins, "Clouds Gather over Novartis As It Battles a Series of Setbacks," Financial Times, April 18, 2016, https://next.ft.com/content/494863e0-03b7-11e6-a70d-4e39ac32c284.

42. Ed Silverman, "Former Pharma Sales Reps Charged with Bribing Docs to Prescribe Opioids," STAT, June 11, 2016, https://www.statnews.com/pharmalot/2016/06/11/fentanyl-opioids-bribes-insys/.

43. Ed Silverman, "Drug Maker Fined for Shorting Supplies of Cancer Drugs in Order to Raise Prices," STAT, October 17, 2016, https://www.statnews.com/pharmalot/2016/10/17/drug-shortage-higher-prices/.

44. Andreas Vilhelmsson, Affiliations: Department of Clinical Sciences, Division of Social Medicine and Global Health, Faculty of Medicine, Malmö University, Lund, Sweden, Department of Gender Studies, Faculty of Social Sciences, Lund University, Lund, Sweden Courtney Davis, and Shai Mulinari, × "Pharmaceutical Industry Off-Label Promotion and Self-Regulation: A Document Analysis of Off-Label Promotion Rulings by the United Kingdom Prescription Medicines Code of Practice Authority 2003–2012," PLoS Medicine 13, no. 1 (2012): e1001945, doi: http://dx.doi.org/10.1371/journal.pmed.1001945.

45. David Evans, "When Drug Makers' Profits Outweigh Penalties," Washington Post, March 21, 2010, http://www.washingtonpost.com/wp-dyn/content/article/2010/03/19/AR2010031905578.html.

46. Ibid.; Fugh-Berman, "How Basic Scientists."

47. Quoted in Evans, "When Drug Makers' Profits Outweigh Penalties."

48. Ravi Katari and Dean Baker, Patent Monopolies and the Costs of Mismarketing Drugs, Center for Economic and Policy Research, 2015, http://cepr.net/documents/publications/mismarketing-drugs-2015-04.pdf.

49. Goldacre, Bad Pharma, 345.

50. Ibid.; Public Citizen, "Pharmaceutical Industry"; Almashat et al., Rapidly Increasing Criminal and Civil Penalties, 17.

51. Fugh-Berman, "How Basic Scientists," 3.

52. Reinhard Angelmar, Sarah Angelmar, and Liz Kane, "Building Strong Condition Brands," Journal of Medical Marketing 7, no. 4 (2007): 341–51, doi: 10.1057/palgrave.jmm.5050101.

53. Antonie Meixel, Elena Yanchar, and Adriane Fugh-Berman, "Hypoactive Sexual Desire Disorder: Inventing a Disease to Sell Low Libido," Journal of Medical Ethics 41, no. 10 (2015): 859–62, doi: 10.1136/medethics-2014-102596.

54. Alan Schwarz, ADHD NATION: Children, Doctors, Big Pharma, and the Making of an American Epidemic (New York: Scribner, 2016); Adam Gaffney, "How ADHD Was Sold," New Republic, September 23, 2016, https://newrepublic.com/article/137066/adhd-sold.

55. Ian Sample, "Viagra: The Profitable Pill," Guardian, November 16, 2009, http://www.theguardian.com/business/2009/nov/16/viagra-pfizer-drug-pill-profit.

56. Meixel, Yanchar, and Berman, "Hypoactive Sexual Desire Disorder."

57. Ibid.

58. Ibid.

59. Ibid.

60. Quoted in Stephanie Strom and Matt Fleischer-Black, "Drug Maker's Vow to Donate Cancer Medicine Falls Short," New York Times, June 5, 2003, http://www.nytimes.com/2003/06/05/business/drug-maker-s-vow-to-donate-cancer-medicine-falls-short.html.

61. Ibid.

62. Ibid.; Lisa Schencker, "Lifesavers or Kickbacks? Critics Say Patient-Assistance Programs Help Keep Drug Prices High," Modern Healthcare, March 7, 2015, http://www.modernhealthcare.com/article/20150307/MAGAZINE/303079980.

63. U.S. Department of Health and Human Services, "Prescription Drugs: Innovation, Spending, and Patient Access," Report to Congress, December 7, 2016, http://apps.who.int/medicinedocs/documents/s23128en/s23128en.pdf, 13, 99.

64. Schencker, "Lifesavers or Kickbacks?"

65. Benjamin Elgin and Robert Langreth, "How Big Pharma Uses Charity Programs to Cover for Drug Price Hikes," Bloomberg News, May 19, 2016, http://www.bloomberg.com/news/articles/2016-05-19/the-real-reason-big-pharma-wants-to-help-pay-for-your-prescription.

66. Ben Elgin and Robert Langreth, "Celgene Accused of Using Charities 'Scheme' to Gain Billions," Bloomberg, August 1, 2016,, http://www.bloomberg.com/news/articles/2016-08-01/celgene-accused-of-using-charities-in-scheme-to-gain-billions.

67. Brian Faler, "Obama Blasts 'Corporate Deserters,'" Politico, July 24, 2014, http://www.politico.com/story/2014/07/obama-corporate-deserters-taxes-109357.

68. John Cassidy, "The Pfizer-Allergan Merger Is a Disgrace," New Yorker, November 23, 2015, http://www.newyorker.com/news/john-cassidy/the-pfizer-allergan-merger-is-a-disgrace.

69. Richard Rubin, "U.S. Companies Are Stashing $2.1 Trillion Overseas to Avoid Taxes," Bloomberg Business, March 4, 2015, http://www.bloomberg.com/news/articles/2015-03-04/u-s-companies-are-stashing-2-1-trillion-overseas-to-avoid-taxes; Engelberg, "How Government Policy."

70. Andrew Pollack, "Drug Patents Held Overseas Can Pare Makers' Tax Bills," New York Times, September 29, 2014, http://www.nytimes.com/2014/09/30/business/patents-put-overseas-can-pare-tax-bills.html?hp&action=click&pgtype.

71. In Americans for Tax Fairness, "New Report: Taxpayer-Supported Gilead Sciences Is Price Gouging the Public Then Dodging Taxes," 2016, http://www.americansfortaxfairness.org/new-report-taxpayer-supported-gilead-sciences-is-price-gouging-the-public-then-dodging-taxes-on-the-huge-profits/.

9. Medicines Are Priced at Whatever the Market Will Bear

1. Andrew Pollack, "Drug Goes from $13.50 a Tablet to $750, Overnight," New York Times, September 20, 2015, http://www.nytimes.com/2015/09/21/business/a-huge-overnight-increase-in-a-drugs-price-raises-protests.html.

2. Heather Long and Matt Egan, "Meet the Guy behind the $750 AIDS Drug," CNN Money, September 22, 2015, http://money.cnn.com/2015/09/22/investing/aids-drug-martin-shkreli-750-cancer-drug; Brett LoGiurato, "Donald Trump Trashes Former Hedge-Fund Guy Who Jacked Up Drug Price: 'He Looks like a Spoiled Brat,'" Business Insider, September 23, 2015, http://www.businessinsider.com/donald-trump-martin-shkreli-daraprim-drug-cost-2015-9.

3. Quoted in Doni Bloomfield, "Drug CEO Targeted by Clinton Is Criticized by Drug Lobby," Bloomberg, September 22, 2015, http://www.bloomberg.com/news/articles/2015-09-22/big-pharma-lobby-group-forswears-drugmaker-targeted-by-clinton.

4. Ibid.

5. Quoted in Robert Langreth and Rebecca Spalding, "Shrkeli Was Right: Everyone's Hiking Drug Prices," Bloomberg, February 2, 2016, http://www.bloomberg.com/news/articles/2016-02-02/shrkeli-not-alone-in-drug-price-spikes-as-skin-gel-soars-1-860.

6. Aaron S. Kesselheim, Jerry Avorn, and Ameet Sarpatwari, "The High Cost of Prescription Drugs in the United States Origins and Prospects for Reform," Journal of the American Medical Association 316, no. 8 (August 23/30, 2016): 858–71, doi:10.1001/jama.2016.11237.

7. "Billion Dollar Babies: The High Cost of R&D Is Used to Explain Why Drugs Giants Merge, and Why They Must Charge High Prices. The Reality Is Somewhat Different," Economist, November 28, 2015, http://www.economist.com/news/business/21679203-high-cost-rd-used-explain-why-drugs-giants-merge-and-why-they-must-charge.

8. Ed Silverman, "NIH Asked to Fight Price Gouging by Overriding Drug Patents," STAT, January 11, 2016, http://www.statnews.com/pharmalot/2016/01/11/nih-drug-costs-patents/; "U.S. Inflation Calculator: Historical Inflation Rates: 1914–2016," Coin News Media Group, accessed June 12, 2016, http://www.usinflationcalculator.com/inflation/historical-inflation-rates/.

9. Langreth and Spalding, "Shrkeli Was Right."

10. Cynthia Koons, "Pfizer Raised Prices on 133 Drugs This Year, and It's Not Alone," Bloomberg News, October 2, 2015, http://www.bloomberg.com/news/articles/2015-10-02/pfizer-raised-prices-on-133-drugs-this-year-and-it-s-not-alone.

11. Ed Silverman, "CMS Official Says Drug Costs Are 'Unsustainable and There Are Too Many 'Bad Actors,'" STAT, November 7, 2016, https://www.statnews.com/pharmalot/2016/11/07/medicare-medicaid-drug-prices/.

12. U.S. Department of Health and Human Services, "Report to Congress: Prescription Drugs: Innovation, Spending, and Patient Access," December 7, 2016, http://apps.who.int/medicinedocs/documents/s23128en/s23128en.pdf, 27.

13. Marie-Paule Kieny, "A Comprehensive and Fair Solution to the Price of Medicines," Huffington Post, June 28, 2016, http://www.huffingtonpost.com/mariepaule-kieny/a-comprehensive-and-fair-_b_10695814.html.

14. Jonathan D. Rockoff, "5 Things to Know about How Drug Prices Are Set," Wall Street Journal (blog), December 8, 2015, http://blogs.wsj.com/briefly/2015/12/08/5-things-to-know-about-how-drug-prices-are-set/; Orrin G, Hatch and Ron Wyden, "Wyden-Grassley Sovaldi Investigation Finds Revenue-Driven Pricing Strategy behind $84,000 Hepatitis Drug," U.S. Senate Committee on Finance, 114th Congress, 1st Sess., Washington, DC, 2015, http://www.finance.senate.gov/ranking-members-news/wyden-grassley-sovaldi-investigation-finds-revenue-driven-pricing-strategy-behind-84-000-hepatitis-drug.

15. Sarah Karlin-Smith, "Price Spikes for Lifesaving Drug," Politico, May 16, 2015, http://www.politico.com/story/2016/05/drug-prices-addiction-223192.

16. Jonathan D. Rockoff, "How Pfizer Set the Cost of Its New Drug at $9,850 a Month," Wall Street Journal, December 9, 2015, http://www.wsj.com/articles/the-art-of-setting-a-drug-price-1449628081.

17. Ben Hirschler, "Exclusive: Americans Overpaying Hugely for Cancer Drugs—Study," Reuters, September 22, 2015, http://www.reuters.com/article/us-health-pharmaceuticals-cancer-usa-idUSKCN0RM1EC20150922.

18. Ibid.; Gregg Gonsalves, "Martin Shkreli Is Just a Tiny Part of a Huge Problem," Nation, September 25, 2015, http://www.thenation.com/article/martin-shkreli-is-just-a-tiny-part-of-a-huge-problem/.

19. Hatch and Wyden, "Wyden-Grassley Sovaldi Investigation."

20. Andrew Hill, Saye Khoo, Joe Fortunak, Bryony Simmons, and Nathan Ford, "Minimum Costs for Producing Hepatitis C Direct-Acting Antivirals for Use in Large-Scale Treatment Access Programs in Developing Countries," Clinical Infectious Diseases 58, no. 7 (2014): 928–36, doi: 10.1093/cid/ciu012.

21. Robert Langreth, "How Gilead Priced Its $20 Million Blockbuster," Bloomberg, December 10, 2015, http://www.bloomberg.com/news/articles/2015-12-10/behind-the-1-000-pill-a-formula-for-profits-inside-gilead.

22. Ibid.

23. Hatch and Wyden, "Wyden-Grassley Sovaldi Investigation."

24. Quoted in Langreth, "How Gilead Priced."

25. Hatch and Wyden, "Wyden-Grassley Sovaldi Investigation."

26. Médecins Sans Frontières/Doctors Without Borders, The Right Shot: Bringing Down Barriers to Affordable and Adapted Vaccines, 2nd ed. (Geneva: MSF Access Campaign, January, 16, 2015), 4, http://www.doctorswithoutborders.org/article/right-shot-bringing-down-barriers-affordable-and-adapted-vaccines-2nd-edition.

27. Ibid., 4, 10, 25.

28. Ibid., 4, 10, 18.

29. Ibid., 17.

30. Ibid., 8, 16, 25.

31. Ibid., 4.

32. Médecins Sans Frontières/Doctors Without Borders, "MSF Welcomes Pfizer's Pneumonia Vaccine Price Reduction For Children in Humanitarian Emergencies," November 15,

2016, https://www.msf.org.au/article/project-news/msf-welcomes-pfizer%E2%80%99s-pneumo
nia-vaccine-price-reduction-children-humanitarian.

33. Langreth and Spalding, "Shrkeli Was Right."

34. Katie Thomas, "Valeant Pharmaceuticals Expands Drug Discount Offer after Criticism," New York Times, May 16, 2016, http://www.nytimes.com/2016/05/17/business/vale
ant-pharmaceuticals-expands-drug-discount-offer-after-criticism.html?_r=0. For a discussion
of the limited impact of such discounts, see Ariana Eunjung Cha, "Why the New EpiPen Cou-
pons Are More about Helping the Company than Helping You," Washington Post, August 26,
2016, https://www.washingtonpost.com/news/to-your-health/wp/2016/08/26/why-the-new-
epipen-coupons-are-more-about-helping-the-company-than-helping-you/?postshare=39614
72255394757&tid=ss_mail.

35. Ed Silverman, "Huge Valeant Price Hike on Lead Poisoning Drug Causes Anger,"
STAT, October 11, 2016, https://www.statnews.com/pharmalot/2016/10/11/valeant-drug-
prices-lead-poisoning/.

36. Ibid.; Koons, "Pfizer Raised Prices."

37. "UK Watchdog Accuses Pfizer of Inflating Anti-Epilepsy Drug Price," Financial Times,
August 6, 2015, http://www.ft.com/intl/cms/s/0/2f32a6e6-3c20-11e5-8613-07d16aad2152.
html.

38. Koons, "Pfizer Raised Prices."

39. Ibid.,; Langreth and Spalding, "Shrkeli Was Right"; Michelle Andrews, "People with
Diabetes Are Facing Rising Prices for Lifesaving Drugs," Washington Post, August 24, 2015,
http://www.washingtonpost.com/national/health-science/people-with-diabetes-are-facing-ris
ing-prices-for-lifesaving-drugs/2015/08/24/dec2abd8-476f-11e5-8e7d-9c033e6745d8_story.
html.

40. Langreth and Spalding, "Shrkeli Was Right"; Jonathan D. Rockoff, "Rising Drug Costs
to Be in Focus at Congressional Heating, " Wall Street Journal, December 5, 2015, http://www.
wsj.com/articles/rising-drug-costs-to-be-in-focus-at-congressional-hearing-1449311407.

41. Médecins Sans Frontières/Doctors Without Borders, "First New TB Drugs in Half a
Century Reach Just 2% of People Who Need Them," news release December 3, 2015, http://
www.msfaccess.org/about-us/media-room/press-releases/first-new-tb-drugs-half-century-
reach-just-2-people-who-need-them.

42. Keith Bradsher and Edmund Andrews, "U.S. Says Bayer Will Cut Cost of Its Anthrax
Drug," New York Times, October 24, 2001, http://www.nytimes.com/2001/10/24/business/a-
nation-challenged-cipro-us-says-bayer-will-cut-cost-of-its-anthrax-drug.html.

43. Kei Research, "KEI Research Note: Recent United States Compulsory Licenses,"
March 7, 2014, http://keionline.org/sites/default/files/Annex_A_US_Compulsory_Licenses_
7Mar2014_8_5x11.pdf, 1–2.

44. Peter B. Bach, Leonard B. Saltz, and Robert Wittes, "In Cancer Care, Cost Matters"
New York Times, October 15, 2012, http://www.nytimes.com/2012/10/15/opinion/a-hospi
tal-says-no-to-an-11000-a-month-cancer-drug.html?_r=0; Ellen t'Hoen; "Access to Cancer
Treatment: A Study of Medicine Pricing Issues with Recommendations for Improving Access
to Cancer Medication," Oxfam, February 2015, https://www.oxfam.org/sites/www.oxfam.
org/files/file_attachments/rr-access-cancer-treatment-inequality-040215-en.pdf, 5.

45. Quoted in Hatch and Wyden, "Wyden-Grassley Sovaldi Investigation."

10. Pharmaceutical Corporations Reap History-Making Profits

1. Richard Anderson, "Pharmaceutical Industry Gets High on Fat Profits," BBC News,
November 6, 2014, http://www.bbc.com/news/business-28212223; World Health Organization, "Trade, Foreign Policy, Diplomacy, and Health: Pharmaceutical Industry," http://

www.who.int/trade/glossary/story073/en/ (page no longer available but information is at Rufus Polluck [blog], May 29, 2016, http://rufuspollock.org/2016/05/29/strong-words-from-who-on-pharma-industry/); Matt Krantz, "Mylan Isn't Alone: 11 Drugmakers with Off-the-Charts Pricing Power," USA Today, August 25, 2016, http://www.usatoday.com/story/money/markets/2016/08/25/mylan-not-only-drugmaker-big-profit-margins/89302124/.

2. Alfred Engelberg, "How Government Policy Promotes High Drug Prices," Health Affairs (blog), October 29, 2015, http://healthaffairs.org/blog/2015/10/29/how-govern ment-policy-promotes-high-drug-prices/Congress of the United States Congressional Bud-get Office, Research and Development in the Pharmaceutical Industry, 44 (2006), https://www.cbo.gov/sites/default/files/109th-congress-2005-2006/reports/10-02-drugr-d.pdf. Alfred Engelberg, "Memo to the President: The Pharmaceutical Monopoly Adjustment Act of 2017," Health Affairs Blog, September 13, 2016, http://healthaffairs.org/blog/2016/09/13/memo-to-the-president-the-pharmaceutical-monopoly-adjustment-act-of-2017/.

3. Mariana Mazzucato, The Entrepreneurial State: Debunking Public vs. Private Sector Myths (New York: Public Affairs, 2015), 203.

4. Anderson, "Pharmaceutical Industry"; Lotti Rutter, "Treatment Action, Campaign_A," United Nations Secretary-General's High-Level Panel on Access to Medicines, February 28, 2016, http://www.unsgaccessmeds. org/inbox/2016/2/28/lotti-rutter; Liyan Chen, "The Most Profitable Industries in 2016," Forbes, December 21, 2015, www.forbes.com/.../2015/12/21/the-most-profitable-industries-in-2016.

5. "Too Much of a Good Thing," Economist, March 16, 2016, http://www.economist.com/news/briefing/21695385-profits-are-too-high-america-needs-giant-dose-competition-too-much-good-thing. According to the article, "abnormal profits come from the health-care industry, where a cohort of pharmaceutical and medical-equipment firms make aggregate returns on capital of 20–50%. The industry is riddled with special interests and is governed by patent rules that allow firms temporary monopolies on innovative new drugs and inventions."

6. Anderson, "Pharmaceutical Industry"; Engelberg, "How Government Policy."

7. Médecins Sans Frontières/Doctors Without Borders, "Access Campaign: MSF Launches Global Action against Pfizer and GlaxoSmithKline to Cut the Price of the Pneumonia Vaccine," press release, November 12, 2015, http://www.msfaccess.org/about-us/media-room/press-releases/msf-launches-global-action-against-pfizer-and-glaxosmith kline-cut; James Hamblin, "Why Doctors Without Borders Refused a Million Free Vac-cines," Atlantic, October 14, 2016, http://www.theatlantic.com/health/archive/2016/10/doctors-with-borders/503786/.

8. Andrew Powaleney, "Fact Check Friday: The Truth about Industry's Role in R&D," PhRMA, The Catalyst, October 23, 2015, http://catalyst.phrma.org/fact-check-friday-the-truth-about-industrys-role-in-r-and-d.

9. John Carey and Amy Barrett, "Drug Prices: What's Fair?" Bloomberg, December 10, 2001, http://www.bloomberg.com/news/articles/2001-12-09/drug-prices-whats-fair.

10. Mazzucato, Entrepreneurial State, 32–33.

11. William Lazonick, "Profits without Prosperity," Harvard Business Review, September, 2014, https://hbr.org/2014/09/profits-without-prosperity. Stock buybacks are now a com-mon occurrence among large corporations even outside the pharmaceutical industry. Over the decade 2003–2012, the companies in the S&P 500 index spent more than half their earnings buying back their own stock.)

12. Ibid.

13. "Pfizer Hikes Prices for over 100 Drugs on January 1," Reuters, January 8, 2016, http://www.nbcnews.com/business/business-news/pfizer-hikes-prices-over-100-drugs-january-1-n493281.

14. Quoted in Robert Langreth, "Pfizer Announces New $10 Billion Share Repurchase Program," Bloomberg, December 12, 2011, http://www.bloomberg.com/news/articles/2011-12-12/pfizer-sets-10-billion-share-buyback-program-boosts-quarterly-dividend.

15. Sean Williams, "The Highest Paid CEOs in Pharma," Motley Fool, June 6, 2015, http://www.fool.com/investing/general/2015/06/06/the-highest-paid-ceos-in-pharma.aspx.

16. Lazonick, "Profits without Prosperity."

17. Ethan Rome, "Big Pharma CEOs Rake in $1.57 Billion in Pay," The Blog, Huffington Post, May 8, 2013, http://www.huffingtonpost.com/ethan-rome/big-pharma-ceo-pay_b_3236641.html.

18. Matt Krantz, "Drug Prices Are High. So Are CEO's Pay," USA Today, August 26, 2016, http://www.usatoday.com/story/money/markets/2016/08/26/drug-money-pharma-ceos-paid-71-more/89369152/; Williams, "Highest Paid CEOs in Pharma"; Dan Munro, "Pharma Trumps All Healthcare Sectors in Executive Compensation," Forbes, May 26, 2015, http://www.forbes.com/sites/danmunro/2015/05/26/pharma-trumps-all-healthcare-sectors-in-executive-compensation/#36305d6b1e47.

19. Victor Roy and Lawrence King, "Betting on Hepatitis C: How Financial Speculation in Drug Development Influences Access to Medicines," BMJ 354 (2016): i3718, doi: http://dx.doi.org/10.1136/bmj.i3718.

20. Lazonick, "Profits without Prosperity."

11. The For-Profit Medicine Arguments Are Patently False

1. Richard DeGeorge, "Two Cheers for the Pharmaceutical Industry," in Ethics and the Business of Biomedicine, ed. Denis G. Arnold (Cambridge, UK: Cambridge University Press, 2009).

2. Ibid., 169.

3. Ibid., 195.

4. Ibid.

5. PhRMA, "About PhRMA," http://www.phrma.org/about (accessed June 17, 2016); "Pharmaceutical Research and Manufacturers of America (PhRMA) Biography, ProCon.org, March 24, 2010, http://prescriptiondrugs.procon.org/view.source.php?sourceID=009637 (accessed June 17, 2016).

6. "Pharmaceuticals/Health Products: Top Contributors 2015–2016," OpenSecrets.org, January 22, 2016, http://www.opensecrets.org/lobby/indusclient.php?id=h04.

7. "Pharmaceuticals/Health Products: Industry Profile 2015," OpenSecrets.org, last modified May 16, 2016, http://www.opensecrets.org/industries/indus.php?ind=H04.

8. Ibid.

9. "Pharmaceutical Manufacturing," OpenSecrets.org, last modified May 16, 2016, http://www.opensecrets.org/industries/indus.php?Ind=H4300.

10. Johnson & Johnson, "Our Credo," http://www.jnj.com/sites/default/files/pdf/jnj_our credo_bnglish_us_8.5x11_cmyk.pdf (accessed June 7, 2016).

11. PhRMA, "Partnership for Prescription Assistance," http://www.phrma.org/access/ppa (accessed June 7, 2016).

12. Robert D. McFadden, "Charles Keating, 90, Key Figure in '80s Savings and Loan Crisis, Dies," New York Times, April 2, 2014, https://www.nytimes.com/2014/04/02/business/charles-keating-key-figure-in-the-1980s-savings-and-loan-crisis-dies-at-90.html?_r=1.

13. Public opinion polling suggests that such an innovation-focused message does blunt the desire for significant reform of the current medicines system. Ed Silverman, "Americans Want Price Controls on Drugs, but Worry about Impeding Innovation, Poll Finds," STAT, January 30, 2017, https://www.statnews.com/pharmalot/2017/01/30/drug-prices-innovation/.

14. PhRMA, "Intellectual Property," http://www.phrma.org/innovation/intellectual-property (accessed June 7, 2016).

15. Kristina Lybecker, "The Sticking Point That Shouldn't Be: The Role of Pharmaceutical Patents in the TPP Negotiations," IPWatchdog, August 3, 2015, http://www.ipwatchdog.com/2015/08/03/role-of-pharmaceutical-patents-in-the-tpp-negotiations/id=60283/.

16. Andrew Hill, Saye Khoo, Joe Fortunak, Bryony Simmons, and Nathan Ford, "Minimum Costs for Producing Hepatitis C Direct-Acting Antivirals for Use in Large-Scale Treatment Access Programs in Developing Countries," Clinical Infectious Diseases 58, no. 7 (2014): 928–36, doi: 10.1093/cid/ciu012.

17. U.S. Food and Drug Administration, "Facts about Generic Drugs," last modified June 19, 2015, http://www.fda.gov/Drugs/ResourcesForYou/Consumers/BuyingUsingMedicineSafely/UnderstandingGenericDrugs/ucm167991.htm#_ftnref3.

18. "History of Medicine Timeline," DatesandEvents.org, http://www.datesandevents.org/events-timelines/10-history-of-medicine-timeline.htm (accessed June 7, 2016); Bhaven N. Sampat and Frank R. Lichtenberg, "What Are the Respective Roles of the Public and Private Sectors in Pharmaceutical Innovation?" Health Affairs 30, no. 2 (2011): 332–39, doi: 10.1377/hlthaff.2009.0917; "Question of Utility: Patents Are Protected by Governments Because They Are Held to Promote Innovation. But There Is Plenty of Evidence That They Do Not," Economist, August 8, 2015, http://www.economist.com/node/21660559?zid=317&ah=8a47fc455a44945580198768fad0fa41; Aaron Kesselheim, Yongtian Tina Tan, and Jerry Avorn, "The Roles of Academia, Rare Diseases, and Repurposing in the Development of the Most Transformative Drugs," Health Affairs 34, no. 2 (2015): 286–93, doi:10.1377/hlthaff.2014.1038.

19. Marcia Angell, The Truth about the Drug Companies: How They Deceive Us and What to Do about It (New York: Random House, 2004), 20.

12. Medicine Patents Are Extended Too Far and Too Wide

1. Melly Alazraki, "The 10 Biggest-Selling Drugs That Are About to Lose Their Patent," Daily Finance, February 27, 2011, http://www.dailyfinance.com/2011/02/27/top-selling-drugs-are-about-to-lose-patent-protection-ready/#sthash.Ip9RmYzf.dpuf; Médecins Sans Frontières/Doctors Without Borders, Untangling the Web of ARV Price Reductions, 10 (2012), https://www.msfaccess.org/sites/default/files/MSF_assets/HIV_AIDS/Docs/AIDS_report_UTW15_BNG_2012.pdf; Melissa J. Barber, Dzintars Gotham, and Andrew Hill, "Potential Price Reductions for Cancer Medicines on the WHO Essential Medicines List," January 2017, https://www.researchgate.net/publication/313064230_Potential_price_reductions_for_cancer_medicines_on_the_WHO_Essential_Medicines_List.

2. Bloomberg News, "Schering-Plough Hurt by Competition to Claritin," New York Times, March 6, 2003, http://www.nytimes.com/2003/03/06/business/company-news-schering-plough-hurt-by-competition-to-claritin.html; "Eli Lilly Gets Prozac Blues," CNN Money, August 9, 2000, http://money.cnn.com/2000/08/09/companies/lilly/index.htm.

3. Quoted in John George, "Hurdles Ahead for Cephalon," Philadelphia Business Journal, March 20, 2006, http://www.bizjournals.com/philadelphia/stories/2006/03/20/story1.html.

4. Amy Kapczynski, Chan Park, and Bhaven Sampat, "Polymorphs and Prodrugs and Salts (Oh My!): An Empirical Analysis of "Secondary" Pharmaceutical Patents," PLoS ONE 7, no. 12 (2012): e49470t, doi: http://dx.doi.org/10.1371/journal.pone.0049470; Carlos M. Correa, "Pharmaceutical Innovation, Incremental Patenting, and Compulsory Licensing," Research Paper no. 41, South Centre, Geneva, September 2011, 5, http://thaipublica.org/wp-content/uploads/2011/12/RP-41-Pharm-CompLice-CCorrea.pdf; European Commission,

"Antitrust: Shortcomings in Pharmaceutical Sector Require Further Action," news release, July 8, 2009, http://europa.eu/rapid/press-release_IP-09-1098_bn.htm?locale=en.

5. Kapczynski et al.

6. Lotti Rutter, Mary-Jane Matsolo, and Catherine Tomlinson, "Reforming South Africa's Patent Laws to Promote Access to Medicines: An Activist Guide to the Fix the Patent Laws Campaign," Treatment Action Campaign February 14, 2014, http://www.tac.org.za/sites/default/files/publications/2014-02-14/Fix_The_Patent_Laws_Activist_Guide.pdf.

7. Correa, "Pharmaceutical Innovation": PhRMA, "Intellectual Property," http://www.phrma.org/innovation/intellectual-property (accessed June 7, 2016).

8. Els Torreele, "Only a Radical Overhaul Can Reclaim Medicines for the Public Interest," PLoS (blog), October 13, 2015, http://blogs.plos.org/yoursay/2015/10/13/talking-about-drug-prices-access-to-medicines/. Veronika J. Wirtz, Hans V. Hogerzeil, Andrew L. Gray, Maryam Bigdeli, Cornelis P. de Joncheere, Margaret A. Ewen, Martha Gyansa-Lutterodt, Sun Jing, Vera L. Luiza, Regina M. Mbindyo, Helene Möller, Corrina Moucheraud, Bernard Pécoul, Lembit Rägo, Arash Rashidian, Dennis Ross-Degnan, Peter N. Stephens, Yot Teerawattananon, Ellen F. M. 't Hoen, Anita K Wagner, Prashant Yadav, Michael R. Reich, "Essential Medicines for Universal Health Coverage," The Lancet, November 7, 2016, http://yolse.org/wp-content/uploads/2016/11/EssentialMeds.pdf, 60.

At the time of this book's writing, billions are being spent by the pharmaceutical corporations Merck and AbbVie, among others, in the quest to grab some of the lucrative market for hepatitis C treatments that mimic the impact of Gilead Sciences' Sovaldi, discussed in chapter 1. Allison Gatlin, "Gilead 'Paralyzed' On Likely Hepatitis C Share Loss to AbbVie, Merck," Investor's Business Daily News, September 27, 2016, http://www.investors.com/news/technology/gilead-paralyzed-on-likely-hepatitis-c-share-loss-to-abbvie-merck-jj/.

9. Correa, "Pharmaceutical Innovation," 6.

10. Kasia Lipska, "Break Up the Insulin Racket," Sunday Review: Opinion, New York Times, February 20, 2016, http://www.nytimes.com/2016/02/21/opinion/sunday/break-up-the-insulin-racket.html.

11. Carolyn Johnson, "Why Treating Diabetes Keeps Getting More Expensive," Washington Post, October 31, 2016, https://www.washingtonpost.com/news/wonk/wp/2016/10/31/why-insulin-prices-have-kept-rising-for-95-years/?postshare=5051478042695109&tid=ss_mail&utm_term=.1d351aa3da55.

12. Lydia Ramsey, "A 93-Year-Old Drug That Can Cost More Than a Mortgage Payment Tells Us Everything That's Wrong With American Healthcare," Business Insider, September 16, 2016, http://www.businessinsider.com/insulin-prices-increase-2016-9.

13. U.S. Food and Drug Administration, "Frequently Asked Questions on Patents and Exclusivity," last modified July 8, 2014, http://www.fda.gov/Drugs/DevelopmentApproval Process/ucm079031.htm#How long is exclusivity granted for?.

14. Sandeep Kishore, Kavitha Kolappa, Jordan D. Jarvis, Paul H. Park, Rachel Belt, Thirukumaran Balasubramaniam, and Rachel Kiddell-Monroe, "Overcoming Obstacles to Enable Access to Medicines for Noncommunicable Diseases in Poor Countries," Health Affairs 34, no. 9 (2015): 1573, doi: 10.1377/hlthaff.2015.0375.

15. Aaron Kesselheim and Daniel Solomon, "Incentives for Drug Development: The Curious Case of Colchicines," New England Journal of Medicine 362 (2010): 2045–47, http://www.nejm.org/doi/full/10.1056/NEJMp1003126.

16. U.S. Office of Management and Budget, The President's Budget for Fiscal Year 2016 (Washington, DC: U.S. Government Publishing Office, 2016), https://www.whitehouse.gov/sites/default/files/omb/budget/fy2016/assets/budget.pdf.

17. Correa, "Pharmaceutical Innovation," 5.

18. Quoted in Andrew Pollack, "Makers of Humira and Enbrel Using New Drug Patents to Delay Generic Versions," New York Times, July 15, 2016, http://www.nytimes.com/2016/07/16/business/makers-of-humira-and-enbrel-using-new-drug-patents-to-delay-generic-versions.html?hpw&rref=health&action=click&pgtype=Homepage&module=well-region&region=bottom-well&WT.nav=bottom-well&_r=0.

19. Peter Loftus, "Panel Recommends FDA Approval of Remicade Knockoff," Wall Street Journal, February 10, 2016, http://www.wsj.com/articles/panel-recommends-fda-approval-of-remicade-knockoff-1455057993.

20. Ron Bouchard, Richard W. Hawkins, Robert Clark, Reidar Hagtvedt, and Jamil Sawani, "Empirical Analysis of Drug Approval: Drug Patenting Linkage for High Value Pharmaceuticals," Northwestern Journal of Technology and Intellectual Property 8, no. 2 (2010): 227, http://scholarlycommons.law.northwestern.edu/cgi/viewcontent.cgi?article=1102&context=njtip.

21. Michele Boldrin and David K. Levine, Against Intellectual Monopoly (New York: Cambridge University Press, 2008), 11.

22. Zachary Roth, "Drug-Makers Paying Off Competitors to Keep Cheap Generics off Market," TPM Muckracker, Talking Points Memo, December 2, 2009, http://talkingpointsmemo.com/muckraker/drug-makers-paying-off-competitors-to-keep-cheap-generics-off-market.

23. Jon Leibowitz, " 'Pay-for-Delay' Settlements in the Pharmaceutical Industry: How Congress Can Stop Anticompetitive Conduct, Protect Consumers = Wallets, and Help Pay for Health Care Reform (the $35 Billion Solution)," June 23, 2009, transcript, Federal Trade Commission, Center for American Progress, June 23, 2009, https://www.ftc.gov/sites/default/files/documents/public_statements/pay-delay-settlements-pharmaceutical-industry-how-congress-can-stop-anticompetitive-conduct-protect/090623payfordelayspeech.pdf.

24. FTC v. Actavis, Inc., 133 S. Ct. 2223 (U.S. 2013).

25. Leibowitz, " 'Pay-for-Delay' Settlements," 5.

26. U.S. Food and Drug Administration, "Generic Competition and Drug Prices," last modified May 13, 2015, http://www.fda.gov/AboutFDA/CentersOffices/OfficeofMedicalProductsandTobacco/CDER/ucm129385.htm.

27. Kapczynski, Park, and Sampat, "Polymorphs and Prodrugs and Salts."

28. Leibowitz, " 'Pay-for-Delay' Settlements," 1–2.

13. Patent Protectionism Stunts the Development of New Medicines

1. PhRMA, "Intellectual Property," http://www.phrma.org/innovation/intellectual-property (accessed June 7, 2016).

2. Michele Boldrin and David K. Levine, "The Case against Patents," Working Paper no. 2012-035A, Federal Reserve Bank of St. Louis, Research Division, June 29, 2012, https://research.stlouisfed.org/wp/2012/2012-035.pdf, 1; Dean Baker, Rigged: How Globalization and the Rules of the Modern Economy Were Structured to Make the Rich Richer (Washington, DC: Center for Economic and Policy Research, 2016), 78–79, 84–91.

3. Michael Heller and Rebecca Eisenberg, "Can Patents Deter Innovation? The Anticommons in Biomedical Research," Science 280, no. 5364 (1998): 698–701, doi: 10.1126/science.280.5364.698.

4. Jennifer C. Molloy, "The Open Knowledge Foundation: Open Data Means Better Science," PLoS Biology 9, no. 12 (2011): e1001195, doi: 10.1371/journal.pbio.1001195.

5. Carlos M. Correa, "Pharmaceutical Innovation, Incremental Patenting, and Compulsory Licensing," Research Paper no. 41, South Centre, Geneva, September 2011, http://thaipublica.org/wp-content/uploads/2011/12/RP-41-Pharm-CompLice-CCorrea.pdf, 2; Adam B. Jaffe and Josh Lerner, Innovation and Its Discontents: How Our Broken Patent System Is

Endangering Innovation and Progress, and What to Do about It (Princeton: Princeton University Press, 2007).

6. Adam B. Jaffe and Josh Lerner, Innovation and Its Discontents: How Our Broken Patent System Is Endangering Innovation and Progress, and What to Do about It (Princeton University Press, 2004), 171.

7. Ron Bouchard, Jamil Sawani, Chris McLelland, and Monika Sawicka, "The Pas de Deux of Pharmaceutical Regulation and Innovation: Who's Leading Whom," Berkeley Technology Law Journal 24, no. 4 (2009): 1461–522, doi: http://dx.doi.org/doi:10.15779/Z38GX1H. The data show that the pharmaceutical industry is leaning away from the development of new drugs and toward incremental changes in existing drugs as a result of firms locking in to discrete rights targets provided for by law.

8. Michele Boldrin and David K. Levine, Against Intellectual Monopoly (New York: Cambridge University Press, 2008), 10.

9. Correa, "Pharmaceutical Innovation," 2.

10. Petra Moser, "Patents and Innovation in Economic History," Social Science Research Network, January 28, 2016, 9–11, doi: http://dx.doi.org/10.2139/ssrn.2712428; Boldrin and Levine, "Case against Patents," 15–16; Josh Lerner, "The Empirical Impact of Intellectual Property Rights on Innovation: Puzzles and Clues," American Economic Review 99, no. 2 (2009): 343–48, http://www.jstor.org/stable/25592422; Boldrin and Levine, Against Intellectual Monopoly, chaps. 9, 4–5.

11. Moser, "Patents and Innovation in Economic History," 16–17; Joerg Baten, Nicola Bianchi, and Petra Moser, "Does Compulsory Licensing Discourage Invention? Evidence from German Patents after World War I," Cato Institute, October 28, 2015, http://www.cato.org/publications/research-briefs-economic-policy/does-compulsory-licensing-discourage-invention-evidence.

12. Moser, "Patents and Innovation in Economic History," 8.

13. Heidi L. Williams, "Intellectual Property Rights and Innovation: Evidence from the Human Genome," Journal of Political Economy 121 (2013), http://economics.mit.edu/files/8647.

14. UN Secretary-General and Co-Chairs of the High-Level Panel, "Final Report: United Nations Secretary-General's High-Level Panel on Access to Health Technologies: Promoting Innovation and Access to Health Technologies," September 14, 2016, 22, http://www.unsgaccessmeds.org/final-report.

15. U.S. Constitution. Art. I, § 8.

16. Jürgen Bitzer and Philipp J.H. Schröder, "The Impact of Entry and Competition by Open Source Software on Innovation Activity," in The Economics of Open Source Software Development, ed. Jürgen Bitzer and Philipp J.H. Schröder (Bigley, UK: Emerald Group Publishing, 2006), 228. Bitzer and Schröder differentiate the greater degree of knowledge spillover resulting from open source software compared to proprietary licensed software. This effect is consistent with prior research measuring the innovative value of open access to research findings; Fiona Murray, Philippe Aghion, Mathias Dewatripont, Julian Kolev, and Scott Stern. "Of Mice and Academics: Examining the Effect of Openness on Innovation." National Bureau of Economic Research Working Paper No. 14819, March 2009, http://www.nber.org/papers/w14819.

17. Anton Hughes, "Open Source—Ditching Patents and Copyright for the Greater Good," The Conversation, February 26, 2012, https://theconversation.com/open-source-ditching-patents-and-copyright-for-the-greater-good-5302.

18. Auren Hoffman, "Engineers Are the Best Deal, So Stock Up on Them," TechCrunch, June 23, 2009, http://techcrunch.com/2009/06/23/engineers-are-the-best-deal-so-stock-up-on-them/.

19. Lucas Laursen, "Tropical Disease: A Neglected Cause," Nature 533 (2016): S68–69, doi: 10.1038/533S68a. See also Parker Foundation, "Parker Foundation Invests $250 Million

in Open and Collaborative Cancer Research to Accelerate Innovation," press release, April 13, 2016, http://www.openhealthnews.com/content/parker-foundation-invests-250-million-open-and-collaborative-cancer-research-accelerate-inno.

20. Tatum Anderson, "Can Open-Source Drug Development Deliver?" Lancet 387, no. 10032 (2016): 1983–84, doi: http://dx.doi.org/10.1016/S0140-6736(16)30518-9.

21. Aaron Kesselheim, Yongtian Tina Tan, and Jerry Avorn, "The Roles of Academia, Rare Diseases, and Repurposing in the Development of the Most Transformative Drugs," Health Affairs 34, no. 2 (2015): 286–93, doi:10.1377/hlthaff.2014.1038.

14. Governments, Not Private Corporations, Drive Medicine Innovation

1. John-Arne Rottingen, Sadie Regmi, Mari Eide, Alison J. Young, Roderik F. Viergever, Christine Årdal, Javier Guzman, Danny Edwards, Stephen A. Matlin, and Robert F. Terry, "Mapping of Available Health Research and Development Data: What's There, What's Missing, and What Role Is There for a Global Observatory?" Lancet 382, no. 9900 (2013): 1286–1307.

2. National Institutes of Health, "Budget," last modified April 4, 2016, https://www.nih.gov/about-nih/what-we-do/budget.

3. National Institutes of Health, "Nobel Laureates," last modified October 11, 2016, http://www.nih.gov/about-nih/what-we-do/nih-almanac/nobel-laureates.

4. Nell Henderson and Michael Schrage, "The Roots of Biotechnology: Government R&D Spawns a New Industry," Washington Post, December 16, 1984.

5. U.S. Food and Drug Administration, "Priority Review Process," last modified September 15, 2014, http://www.fda.gov/ForPatients/Approvals/Fast/ucm405405.htm.

6. Bhaven N. Sampat and Frank R. Lichtenberg, "What Are the Respective Roles of the Public and Private Sectors in Pharmaceutical Innovation?" Health Affairs 30, no. 2 (2011): 332–39, doi: 10.1377/hlthaff.2009.0917.

7. Connie Mack, "The Benefits of Medical Research and the Role of the NIH," United States Senate, May 17, 2000, http://www.faseb.org/portals/2/pdfs/opa/2008/nih_research_benefits.pdf.

8. Aaron Kesselheim, Yongtian Tina Tan, and Jerry Avorn, "The Roles of Academia, Rare Diseases, and Repurposing in the Development of the Most Transformative Drugs," Health Affairs 34 no. 2 (2015): 286–93, doi:10.1377/hlthaff.2014.1038; Benjamin Zycher, Joseph A. DiMasi, and Christopher-Paul Milne, "Private Sector Contributions to Pharmaceutical Science: Thirty-Five Summary Case Histories," American Journal of Therapeutics 17 (2010): 101–20.

9. Ashley J. Stevens, Jonathan J. Jensen, Katrine Wyller, Patrick C. Kilgore, Sabarni Chatterjee, and Mark L. Rohrbaugh, "The Role of Public-Sector Research in the Discovery of Drugs and Vaccines," New England Journal of Medicine 364 (2011) : 535–41 doi: 10.1377/hlthaff.2014.1038.

10. James Love, "The U.S. Orphan Drug Tax Credit," Knowledge Ecology International, August 7, 2010, http://www.keionline.org/node/905.

11. Michele Boldrin and David K. Levine, Against Intellectual Monopoly (New York: Cambridge University Press, 2008), 15.

12. Ellen t'Hoen, "Access to Cancer Treatment: A Study of Medicine Pricing Issues with Recommendations for Improving Access to Cancer Medication," Oxfam, February 2015, https://www.oxfam.org/sites/www.oxfam.org/files/file_attachments/rr-access-cancer-treatment-inequality-040215-en.pdf,10.

13. Merrill Goozner, The $800 Million Pill: The Truth behind the Costs of New Drugs (Berkeley: University of California Press, 2004), 157–63; National Cancer Institute, "A Story

of Discovery: Gleevec Transforms Cancer Treatment for Chronic Myelogenous Leukemia," http://www.cancer.gov/research/progress/discovery/gleevec (accessed June 17, 2016).

14. Stevens et al., "Role of Public-Sector Research"; Médecins Sans Frontières/Doctors Without Borders, The Right Shot: Bringing Down Barriers to Affordable and Adapted Vaccines, 2nd ed. (Geneva: MSF Access Campaign, January, 16, 2015), 17, http://www.doctorswithoutborders. org/article/right-shot-bringing-down-barriers-affordable-and-adapted-vaccines-2nd-edition.

15. Marianna Mazzucato, The Entrepreneurial State: Debunking Public vs. Private Sector Myths (London: Anthem Press, 2015), 1.

16. Hiroaki Mitsuya, Kent Weinhold, Robert Yarchoan, Dani Bolognesi, and Samuel Broder, "Credit Government Scientists with Developing Anti-AIDS Drug," Letter to the Editor, New York Times, September 28, 1989, http://www.nytimes.com/1989/09/28/opinion/l-credit-government-scientists-with-developing-anti-aids-drug-015289.html.

17. Peter Drahos and John Braithwaite, "Briefing 32: Who Owns the Knowledge Economy? Political Organising behind TRIPS," The Corner House, September 30, 2004, http://www.thecornerhouse.org.uk/resource/who-owns-knowledge-economy.

18. Mazzucato, Entrepreneurial State, 4, 12, 27.

19. Quoted in James Bennett, " 'We Need an Energy Miracle,' " Atlantic, November 2015, http://www.theatlantic.com/magazine/archive/2015/11/we-need-an-energy-miracle/407881/.

15. Taxpayers and Patients Pay Twice for Patented Medicines

1. David Hammerstein, "It Is Not Healthy: Mending the Broken Medicines Innovation Model" (speech), Trans Atlantic Consumer Dialogue discussion at European Parliament, December 2, 2015, streamovations player, 1:58:17, http://tacd.org/event/it-is-not-healthy-mending-the-broken-medicines-innovation-model/.

2. Bayh-Dole Act, Pub. L. No. 96-517, 94 Stat. 3015-28 (2000) (Bayh-Dole Act, 35 U.S.C. §§200–212 (2000 & Supp. II 2002)).

3. Peter Drahos and John Braithwaite, "Briefing 32: Who Owns the Knowledge Economy? Political Organising behind TRIPS," The Corner House, September 30, 2004, http://www.thecornerhouse.org.uk/resource/who-owns-knowledge-economy.

4. Suzanne Elvidge, "The Strength at The Interface: Academia Meets Biopharma Industry," Life Science Leader, July 31, 2014, http://www.lifescienceleader.com/doc/the-strength-at-the-interface-academia-meets-biopharma-industry-0001.

5. Marcia Angell, The Truth about the Drug Companies: How They Deceive Us and What to Do about It (New York: Random House, 2004), 52–73; Marianna Mazzucato, The Entrepreneurial State: Debunking Public vs. Private Sector Myths (London: Anthem Press, 2015), 11, 30–32.

6. Alfred Engelberg, "How Government Policy Promotes High Drug Prices," Health Affairs (blog), October 29, 2015, http://healthaffairs.org/blog/2015/10/29/how-government-policy-promotes-high-drug-prices/.

7. Andrew Pollack, "Cutting Dosage of Costly Drug Spurs a Debate," New York Times, March 16, 2008, http://www.nytimes.com/2008/03/16/business/16gaucher.html?_r=0.

8. Angell, Truth about the Drug Companies.

9. Ellen t'Hoen, "Access to Cancer Treatment: A Study of Medicine Pricing Issues with Recommendations for Improving Access to Cancer Medication," Oxfam, February 2015, https://www.oxfam.org/sites/www.oxfam.org/files/file_attachments/rr-access-cancer-treatment-inequality-040215-en.pdf, 10.

10. Carolyn Y. Johnson, "Taxpayers Helped Fund This $129,000 Cancer Drug. Should the Government Help Cut the Price?" Wonkblog (blog), Washington Post, January 14, 2016, https://www.washingtonpost.com/news/wonk/wp/2016/01/14/taxpayers-helped-fund-this-129000-cancer-drug-should-the-government-help-cut-the-price/.

11. "Letter from Senator Bernie Sanders to the VA, Asking for Compulsory Licenses on Hepatitis C Drugs," Knowledge Ecology International (blog), May 12, 2015, http://keionline.org/node/2230; Jeffrey Sachs, "The Drug That Is Bankrupting America," The Blog, Huffington Post, February 16, 2015, http://www.huffingtonpost.com/jeffrey-sachs/the-drug-that-is-bankrupt_b_6692340.html.

12. Dean Baker, Rigged: How Globalization and the Rules of the Modern Economy Were Structured to Make the Rich Richer (Washington, DC: Center for Economic and Policy Research, 2016), 77–114.

16. Medicines Are a Public Good

1. Portions of this section were originally published as Fran Quigley, "Corporations Killed Medicine. Here's How to Take It Back," Foreign Policy in Focus, February 5, 2016, http://fpif.org/corporations-killed-medicine-heres-take-back/ (reprinted in Nation, February 12, 2016).

2. Hugh Gravelle and Ray Rees, Microeconomics, 3rd ed. (London: Pearson Education, 2004), 326–28, https://ignorelist.files.wordpress.com/2012/01/microeconomics-gravelle-and-rees.pdf.

3. Thomas Jefferson, "Letter to Isaac McPherson," (August 13, 1813), in Writings of Thomas Jefferson, ed. Henry A. Washington, Vol. 6 (Washington, DC: Taylor & Maury, 1853–1854), 180, 181–82. Another U.S. founding father, Benjamin Franklin, refused to take patents on any of his many inventions, including the Franklin stove. "As we enjoy great advantages from the inventions of others, we should be glad of an opportunity to serve others by any invention of ours, and this we should do freely and generously." Quoted in Walter Isaacson, Benjamin Franklin: An American Life (New York: Simon & Schuster, 2004), 132.

4. Richard Cornes and Todd Sandler, The Theory of Externalities, Public Goods, and Club Goods (Cambridge, UK: Cambridge University Press, 1996), 3–12.

5. Gravelle and Rees, Microeconomics, 319.

6. "World Health Organization Declares Smallpox Eradicated 1980," Public Broadcasting Service, last modified 1998, http://www.pbs.org/wgbh/aso/databank/entries/dm79sp.html.

7. World Health Organization, "Spending on Health: A Global Overview," last modified April 2012, http://www.who.int/mediacentre/factsheets/fs319/en/.

8. Ibid.

9. Ian Bremmer, "These 5 Facts Explain the Obstacles to the Trans-Pacific Partnership," Time, August 7, 2015, http://time.com/3980075/these-5-facts-explain-the-obstacles-to-the-trans-pacific-partnership/. The ten largest pharmaceutical companies in the world are located in the United States and Europe.

10. "EU Debates Biopiracy Law to Protect Indigenous People," Guardian, May 1, 2013, http://www.theguardian.com/global-development/2013/may/01/eu-biopiracy-protect-indigenous-people; Michael Carome, "Unethical Clinical Trials Still Being Conducted in Developing Countries," Huffington Post, December 3, 2014, http://www.huffingtonpost.com/michael-carome-md/unethical-clinical-trials_b_5927660.html.

11. Thomas Pogge, "Harnessing the Power of Pharmaceutical Innovation" in The Power of Pills: Social, Ethical, and Legal Issues in Drug Development, Marketing and Pricing, ed. Jillian Claire Cohen, Patricia Illingworth, and Udo Schuklent (London: Pluto Press 2006), 142–49. According to Pogge, "while such exclusion (of consumers due to high cost of patented product) may be acceptable for other categories of intellectual property (software, films and music), it is morally highly problematic in the case of essential medicines," 144–45. James Love, "Coalition for Affordable T-DM1 Asks the Government to Employ Crown Use

Authority to Lower Price of Expensive Cancer Drug," James Love's Blog, Knowledge Ecology International, September 30, 2015, http://keionline.org/node/2328. Love quotes Susanna Markandya, Barrister: "Our drug system has not been there forever, and it was not chosen because it is the most effective way to make medications. It was chosen because it was the best way for drug companies to make money. An unfortunate side-effect of this system, is that millions of people have died from lack of access to medicines. People everywhere are suffering, simply because of their financial capacity. Is that right? At moments like this, we have the chance to change things, to improve them. It's simply a question of public and political will. We have to ask ourselves 'what sort of world do we want to live in?'"

12. Hans V. Hogerzeil, "Essential Medicines and Human Rights: What Can They Learn from Each Other?" Bulletin of the World Health Organization 84, no. 5 (2006): 371–75, http://www.who.int/bulletin/volumes/84/5/371.pdf; S. Katrina Perehudoff, Richard O. Laing, and Hans V. Hogerzeil, "Access to Essential Medicines in National Constitutions," Bulletin of the World Health Organization 88, no. 11 (2010): 800, doi: 10.2471/BLT.10.078733.

13. Pogge, "Harnessing the Power of Pharmaceutical Innovation"; Michele Boldrin and David K. Levine, Against Intellectual Monopoly (New York: Cambridge University Press, 2008), 16.

14. "Vatican—Nearly 2 Billion People without Access to Basic Medicine" Agenzia Fides, June 9, 2010, http://www.fides.org/en/news/26827-VATICAN_Nearly_2_billion_people_without_access_to_basic_medicine#.Vrjs8jbSk5u; Médecins Sans Frontières /Doctors Without Borders, "Medicine Shouldn't be a Luxury," MSF Access Campaign, 1999, http://www.msfaccess.org/content/medicines-shouldnt-be-luxury.

15. "Scientist Manuel E. Patarroyo," The Other Look of Colombia, http://theotherlookofcolombia.com/patarroyo.html (accessed June 15, 2016).

16. Craig Idlebrook, "Selling a Lifetime of Insulin for $3," Insulin Nation, August 7, 2015, http://insulinnation.com/treatment/medicine-drugs/selling-lifetime-insulin/.

17. Amanda McGowan, "Jonas Salk and the War against Polio," WGBH (blog), May 8, 2014, http://blogs.wgbh.org/innovation-hub/2014/5/8/vaccine-wanted-dead-or-alive/.

18. Quoted in Global Citizen, "Could You Patent the Sun?" YouTube video, 01:02, posted January 29, 2013, https://www.youtube.com/watch?v=erHXKP386Nk.

19. Daniel Callahan, "Medicine and the Market," in Ethics and the Business of Biomedicine, ed. Denis G. Arnold (Cambridge, UK: Cambridge University Press, 2009), 20–34. Here is how Callahan describes the market fallacy in health care: "The market rewards strong, knowledgeable individuals, and tolerates the failure or entrepreneurs and commercial enterprises (and the success of others) as a sign of the potency of competition. But the world of the sick is marked by a loss of strength and independence, by a diminishment of self-management, by a painful dependence on others. Providing the economic and social goods to well manage that combination of human vulnerabilities has not been a mark of the market anywhere, nor is there any reason to suppose they could or would be" (33). Callahan expanded on this theme in Daniel Callahan and Angela Wasunna, Medicine and the Market: Equity vs. Choice (Baltimore: John Hopkins University Press, 2006).

20. Adam Mannan and Alan Story, "Abolishing the Product Patent: A Step Forward for Global Access to Drugs," in Power of Pills: Social, Ethical and Legal Issues in Drug Development, Marketing and Pricing, ed. Jillian Clare Cohen, Patricia Illingworth, and Udo Schüklenk (Ann Arbor, MI: Pluto Press, 2006), 179–89. "[U]ntil very recently few countries recognized pharmaceutical product patents. Pharmaceutical product patents are a recent introduction in many countries, including France [1968], Germany [1968], the Nordic countries [1968], Japan [1976], Switzerland [1978], Italy [1978], Canada [1987], Spain [1992], Thailand [1992], Argentina [2000], and India [2005]" (183). See also Brook Baker and Tenu

Avafia, "The Evolution of IPRs from Humble Beginnings to the Modern Day TRIPS-Plus Era: Implications for Treatment Access," working paper, Third Meeting of the Technical Advisory Group of the Global Commission on HIV and the Law, July 2011, p. 4, http://www.hivlaw commission.org/index.php/working-papers?task=document.viewdoc&id=101; Ellen t'Hoen, The Global Politics of Pharmaceutical Monopoly Power: Drug Patents, Access, Innovation and the Application of the WTO Doha Declaration on TRIPS and Public Health (Diemen, Netherlands: AMB, 2009), 16, 39–40, http://www.msfaccess.org/sites/default/files/MSF_assets/Access/Docs/ACCESS_book_GlobalPolitics_tHoen_BNG_2009.pdf.

21. Lembit Rägo and Budiono Santoso, "Drug Regulation: History, Present, and Future," in Drug Benefits and Risk: International Textbook of Clinical Pharmacology, rev. 2nd ed., ed. Christoffel Josvan Boxtel, Budiono Santoso, and I. Ralph Edwards, chap. 6 (Amsterdam: IOS Press and Uppsala Monitoring Centre, 2008), http://www.who.int/medicines/technical_brief ing/tbs/Drug_Regulation_History_Present_Future.pdf.

22. German Lopez, "After Public Outcry, Pharmaceutical Company to Cut Price of Drug It Hiked by 5,500 Percent," Vox, September 22, 2015, http://www.vox.com/2015/9/22/9375295/turing-daraprim-price-cut.

23. John-Arne Røttingen, Sadie Regmi, Mari Eide, Alison J. Young, Roderik F. Viergever, Christine Årdal, Javier Guzman, Danny Edwards, Stephen A. Matlin, and Robert F. Terry, "Mapping of Available Health Research and Development Data: What's There, What's Missing, and What Role Is There for a Global Observatory?" Lancet 382, no. 990 (2013): 1286–307, doi: http://dx.doi.org/10.1016/S0140-6736(13)61046-6; U.S. Congressional Budget Office, "Prices for Name-Brand Drugs under Selected Federal Programs," June 1, 2005, http://www.cbo.gov/sites/default/files/cbofiles/ftpdocs/64xx/doc6481/06-16prescript drug.pdf, 1.

24. Act Up New York, "The Ashes Action," http://www.actupny.org/diva/synAshes.html (accessed June 15, 2016); Vivienne Walt, "AIDS Drug War Heats Up," Fortune, June 25, 2001, http://archive.fortune.com/magazines/fortune/fortune_archive/2001/06/25/305410/index.htm.

25. The United States President's Emergency Plan for AIDS Relief, "PEPFAR," http://www.pepfar.gov/ (accessed June 15, 2016); The Global Fund, http://www.theglobalfund.org/en/ (accessed June 15, 2016).

26. James Boyle, "Fencing Off Ideas: Enclosure and the Disappearance of the Public Domain," Daedalus 131, no. 2 (2002): 13–25, https://law.duke.edu/boylesite/daedalus.pdf.

27. Karl Marx, Das Kapital (Hamburg: O. Meissner, 1867), 15: 5.

28. Edward P. Thompson, The Making of the English Working Class (London: Gollancz, 1963), 218.

29. Of course, this phenomenon is not limited to the English enclosure movement or the modern pharmaceutical industry. Dr. Martin Luther King warned the United States in 1967 about the dangers of a society where "property rights are considered more important than people." "Beyond Vietnam," speech at Riverside Church, New York, April 1967. And Naomi Klein, activist and author, traces the modern-day environmental crisis to a "privatization of the public sphere." This Changes Everything (New York: Simon & Schuster, 2014), 9, 19.

17. Medicine Patents Are Artificial, Recent, and Government-Created

1. Frank Pager, "The Early Growth and Influence of Intellectual Property," Journal of the Patent Office Society 34, no. 2 (1950):106–40, 111, http://www.compilerpress.ca/Library/Prager%20Early%20Growth%20&%20Influence%20of%20IP%20JPOS%201950.htm.

2. Ibid., 116.

3. Peter Drahos and John Braithwaite, "Briefing 32: Who Owns the Knowledge Economy? Political Organising behind TRIPS," The Corner House, September 30, 2004, http://www.thecornerhouse.org.uk/resource/who-owns-knowledge-economy.

4. Brook Baker and Tenu Avafia, "The Evolution of IPRs from Humble Beginnings to the Modern Day TRIPS-Plus Era: Implications for Treatment Access," working paper, Third Meeting of the Technical Advisory Group of the Global Commission on HIV and the Law, July 2011, 2, http://www.hivlawcommission.org/index.php/working-papers?task=document.viewdoc&id=101.

5. Irene Kosturakis, "Intellectual Property 101," Texas Journal of Business Law 46 (fall 2014): 37, 39.

6. Baker and Avafia, "Evolution of IPRs," 4.

7. Ibid.

8. Carolyn Deere, The Implementation Game: The TRIPS Agreement and the Global Politics of Intellectual Property Reform in Developing Countries (London: Oxford University Press, 2009), 35.

9. Amy Kapczynski, "Harmonization and Its Discontents: A Case Study of TRIPS Implementation in India's Pharmaceutical Sector," California Law Review 97 (2009): 1571, http://papers.ssrn.com/sol3/papers.cfm?abstract_id=1557832.

10. Michele Boldrin and David K. Levine, Against Intellectual Monopoly (New York: Cambridge University Press, 2008), 2.

11. Kapczynski, "Harmonization and Its Discontents."

12. Simon Reid-Henry and Hans Lofgren, "Pharmaceutical Companies Putting Health of World's Poor at Risk," Guardian, July 26, 2012, http://www.theguardian.com/global-development/poverty-matters/2012/jul/26/pharmaceutical-companies-health-worlds-poor-risk. See the conclusion of this book for the critical role that Indian generic antiretroviral drugs played in the struggle to address the HIV/AIDS pandemic at the turn of this century.

13. Drahos and Braithwaite, "Briefing 32."

14. Adam Mannan and Alan Story, "Abolishing the Product Patent: A Step Forward for Global Access to Drugs," in Power of Pills: Social, Ethical and Legal Issues in Drug Development, Marketing and Pricing, ed. Jillian Clare Cohen, Patricia Illingworth and Udo Schüklenk (Ann Arbor, MI: Pluto Press, 2006), 183; Boldrin and Levine, Against Intellectual Monopoly, 3–4.

15. Mannan and Story, "Abolishing the Product Patent"; Boldrin and Levine, Against Intellectual Monopoly.

16. Boldrin and Levine, Against Intellectual Monopoly.

17. Ibid.

18. Baker and Avafia, "Evolution of IPRs," 4.

19. United Nations Human Right Council, 28th Session, "Statement by Ms. Farida Shaheed SPECIAL Rapporteur in the Field of Cultural Rights," March 11, 2015, http://www.ip-watch.org/weblog/wp-content/uploads/2015/03/Statement-SR-cultural-rights-11-March.pdf, 4.

20. Ellen t'Hoen, The Global Politics of Pharmaceutical Monopoly Power: Drug Patents, Access, Innovation and the Application of the WTO Doha Declaration on TRIPS and Public Health (Diemen, Netherlands: AMB, 2009), 40, http://www.msfaccess.org/sites/default/files/MSF_assets/Access/Docs/ACCESS_book_GlobalPolitics_tHoen_BNG_2009.pdf. t'Hoen discusses the early-twentieth-century drug company support for compulsory licensing.

21. Peter Drahos and John Braithwaite, Information Feudalism: Who Owns the Knowledge Economy? (New York: Earthscan, 2007).

22. Ibid.

23. Ibid.

24. Ibid.

25. Alan Beattie, "The Flaws in the Geopolitical case for the TPP," *Financial Times* (blog), March 25, 2015, http://blogs.ft.com/the-world/2015/03/the-flaws-in-the-geopolitical-case-for-the-tpp/. According to Beattie, "It's not clear that a country's affection for the US will increase after being required to rewrite its patent and copyright law every few years on a model dictated by, respectively, the Pharmaceutical Research and Manufacturers of America and the Recording Industry Association of America." See also Benjamin F. Jones and Philip Levy, "What Will the TPP Accomplish?" Kellogg Insight (blog), July 10, 2015, http://insight. kellogg.northwestern.edu/article/what-will-the-tpp-accomplish.

26. Michele Boldrin and David K. Levine, "The Case against Patents," Working Paper no. 2012–035A 1, Federal Reserve Bank of St. Louis, Research Division, June 29, 2012, https://research.stlouisfed.org/wp/2012/2012-035.pdf, 20.

27. Dean Baker, "Prescription Drugs and the Trans-Pacific Partnership: Big Pharma Hit by Skills Shortage," Beat the Press, Center for Economic and Policy Research, March 26, 2016, http://cepr.net/blogs/beat-the-press/prescription-drugs-and-the-trans-pacific-partnership-big-pharma-hit-by-skills-shortage.

28. Quoted in Robert Pear, "Drug Companies Increase Spending to Lobby Congress and Governments,"New York Times, June 1, 2003, http://www.nytimes.com/2003/06/01/national/ 01LOBB.html.

29. Statista, "Top Lobbying Industries in the United States in 2014," http://www.statista. com/statistics/257364/top-lobbying-industries-in-the-us/ (accessed June 15, 2016); "Top Interest Groups Giving to Members of Congress, 2016 Cycle," OpenSecrets.org, http://www.opense crets.org/industries/mems.php (accessed June 15, 2016).

30. Drahos and Braithwaite, "Briefing 32."

31. Ibid.

32. "Identification of Countries That Deny Adequate Protection, or Market Access, for Intellectual Property Rights," 19 U.S.C. A §2242 (2016).

33. Christine Thelen, "Carrots and Sticks: Evaluating the Tools for Securing Successful TRIPS Implementation," Temple Journal of Science, Technology and Environmental Law 24, no. 2 (2005): 519, 524n31 http://www.temple.edu/law/tjstel/2005/fall/v24no2-Thelen.pdf.

34. Drahos and Braithwaite, "Briefing 32." According to Drahos and Braithwaite, "When, on 20 October 1988, the US President imposed US$39 million of tariff increases on Brazilian paper products, non-benezoid drugs and consumer electronic items being imported into the US market, Brazil was faced with a cost-benefit calculation. The cost of not complying with US wishes was roughly equal to the death of their markets in these sectors. At that time, almost one-quarter of Brazilian trade was with the US. . . . In 1996 a USTR [U.S. trade representative] Fact Sheet on Special 301 stated that Brazil had taken 'the admirable step of enacting a modern patent law.'"

35. World Health Organization, "Network for Monitoring the Impact of Globalisation and TRIPS on Access to Medicines," 2002, http://apps.who.int/medicinedocs/pdf/s2284e/ s2284e.pdf, 15.

36. Drahos and Braithwaite, "Briefing 32."

37. World Trade Organization, "Agreement on Trade-Related Aspects of Intellectual Property Rights," April 15, 1994, https://www.wto.org/english/docs_e/legal_e/legal_e.htm# finalact.

38. Edmund J. Pratt, "Intellectual Property Rights and International Trade," Pfizer Forum, 1996, quoted in "WTO Millennium Bug: TNC Control Over Global Trade Politics," Corporate

Europe Observer, no. 4, special WTO edition (1999), http://iatp.org/files/WTO_Millennium_Bug_TNC_Control_over_Global_Tra.htm.

39. World Trade Organization, "Agreement," art. 33.

40. Raymond A. Smith and Patricia D. Siplon, Drugs into Bodies: Global AIDS Treatment Activism (Westport, CT: Praeger, 2006), 51.

18. The United States and Big Pharma Play the Bully in Extending Patents

1. World Trade Organization, "Agreement on Trade-Related Aspects of Intellectual Property," April 15, 1994, art. 6, 31, https://www.wto.org/english/docs_e/legal_e/legal_e.htm#finalact.

2. Duncan Matthews, "WTO Decision on Implementation of Paragraph 6 of the Doha Declaration on the TRIPS Agreement and Public Health: A Solution to the Access to Essential Medicines Problem?" Journal of International Economic Law 7 (2004): 73, 80.

3. Medicines and Related Substances and Control Act of 1997, No. 90 (1997) (South Africa); Pharmaceutical Manufacturers. Association of South Africa v. President of the Republic of South Africa, case no. 4193/98, filed February 18, 1998.

4. DaveDC, "Victory Brunch with John Podesta, in Home of Lobbyist Tony Podesta. For Hillary Clinton," DailyKos, February 21, 2016, http://www.dailykos.com/story/2016/2/21/1488725/-Victory-brunch-with-John-Podesta-in-home-of-lobbyist-Tony-Podesta-For-Hillary-Clinton.

5. Meridith Wadman, "Gore under Fire in Controversy over South African AIDS Drug Law," Nature, June 24, 1999, http://www.nature.com/wcs/b51.html.

6. Brook Baker and Tenu Avafia, "The Evolution of IPRs from Humble Beginnings to the Modern Day TRIPS-Plus Era: Implications for Treatment Access," working paper, Third Meeting of the Technical Advisory Group of the Global Commission on HIV and the Law, July 2011, 11, http://www.hivlawcommission.org/index.php/working-papers?task=document.viewdoc&id=101.

7. WTO, "Agreement," art. 1.

8. Ruth Lopert and Deborah Gleeson, "The High Price of 'Free' Trade: U.S. Trade Agreements and Access to Medicines," Journal of Law, Medicine & Ethics 41, no. 1 (2013): 199–223, doi: 0.1111/jlme.12014.

9. Baker and Avafia, "Evolution of IPRs," 13.

10. Jennryn Wentzler, Mihir Mankad, and Adam Burrowbridge, "Timeline for U.S.-Thailand Compulsory License Dispute," Program on Informational Justice and Intellectual Property, April, 2009, http://infojustice.org/wp-content/uploads/2012/11/pijip-thailand-timeline.pdf.

11. Quoted in Joshua Goodman and Linda A. Johnson "Colombia Battles World's Biggest Drugmaker over Cancer Drug." Associated Press, May 18, 2016, http://bigstory.ap.org/article/622371a73e3f43e197875402ce6449ab/colombia-battles-worlds-biggest-drugmaker-over-cancer-drug.

12. Lopert and Gleeson, "High Price of 'Free' Trade," 201–2.

13. Lisa Forman, "Trading Health for Profit: The Impact of Bilateral and Regional Free Trade Agreements on Domestic Intellectual Property Rules on Pharmaceuticals," in Power of Pills: Social, Ethical and Legal Issues in Drug Development, Marketing and Pricing, ed. Jillian Clare Cohen, Patricia Illingworth, and Udo Schüklenk (Ann Arbor: Pluto Press, 2006), 190–200.

14. Médecins Sans Frontières/Doctors Without Borders, "South Africa Should Override Patent on Key HIV Medicine after Widespread Stock Out Problem," news release, October 27, 2015, http://www.msfaccess.org/about-us/media-room/press-releases/south-africa-should-override-patent-key-hiv-medicine-after.

15. Ellen t'Hoen, "Access to Cancer Treatment: A Study of Medicine Pricing Issues with Recommendations for Improving Access to Cancer Medication," Oxfam, February 2015, https://www.oxfam.org/sites/www.oxfam.org/files/file_attachments/rr-access-cancer-treatment-inequality-040215-en.pdf, 45; Médecins Sans Frontières/Doctors Without Borders, The Right Shot: Bringing Down Barriers to Affordable and Adapted Vaccines, 2nd ed. (Geneva: MSF Access Campaign, January, 16, 2015), 4, http://www.doctorswithoutborders.org/article/right-shot-bringing-down-barriers-affordable-and-adapted-vaccines-2nd-edition.

16. Brand India Pharm, "Indian Pharma Sector to Create More Jobs," Pharma Trends, December 10, 2013, http://www.brandindiapharma.in/pharmaceutical-industry-trends/indian-pharma-sector-to-create-more-jobs.

17. t'Hoen, "Access to Cancer Treatment," 46; Subhashini Chandrasekharan, "Intellectual Property Rights and Challenges for Development of Affordable Human Papillomavirus, Rotavirus and Pneumococcal Vaccines: Patent Landscaping and Perspectives of Developing Country Vaccine Manufacturers," Vaccine 33, no. 46 (2015): 6366–70, doi:10.1016/j.vaccine.2015.08.063.

18. is in Article 9.1(f), New Zealand Foreign Affairs and Trade, U.S. International Trade Administration, "2016 Top Markets Report Pharmaceuticals," 2016, http://trade.gov/top markets/pdf/Pharmaceuticals_Executive_Summary.pdf, 4.

19. Médecins Sans Frontières/Doctors Without Borders, Right Shot, 4.

20. t'Hoen, "Access to Cancer Treatment," 46; Médecins Sans Frontières/Doctors Without Borders, "South Africa Should Override Patent."

21. Médecins Sans Frontières/Doctors Without Borders, "Don't Shut Down the Pharmacy of the Developing World: Hands Off Our Medicines," http://www.msf.org/en/hands-our-medicines (accessed June 15, 2016).

22. "Timeline: How the Anthrax Terror Unfolded," National Public Radio, February 15, 2011, http://www.npr.org/2011/02/15/93170200/timeline-how-the-anthrax-terror-unfolded.

23. Keith Bradsher, "The Antibiotic; Bayer Insists Cipro Supply Is Sufficient; Fights Generic," New York Times, October 21, 2001, http://www.nytimes.com/2001/10/21/us/nation-challenged-antibiotic-bayer-insists-cipro-supply-sufficient-fights.html.

24. Quoted in Associated Press, "Government Threatens to Suspend Patent on Cipro," USA Today, October 23, 2001, http://usatoday30.usatoday.com/news/attack/2001/10/23/anthrax-cipro.htm.

25. Keith Bradsher and Edmund Andrews, "A Nation Challenged: U.S. Says Bayer Will Cut Cost of Its Anthrax Drug." New York Times, October 24, 2001, http://www.nytimes.com/2001/10/24/business/a-nation-challenged-cipro-us-says-bayer-will-cut-cost-of-its-anthrax-drug.html.

26. Ibid.

27. "Patent Protection vs. Public Health," Lancet 358, no. 9293 (2011): 1563, doi: 10.1016/S0140-6736(01)06633-8.

28. Smith and Siplon, Drugs into Bodies, 117.

29. Berne Convention Implementation Act of 1988, Pub. L. No. 100–568, 102 Stat. 2853 (1988).

30. Schillinger v. United States, 155 U.S. 163, 168 (1894).

31. Quoted in Daniel Okrent, "'The Wright Brothers,' by David McCullough," Sunday Book Review, New York Times, May 4, 2015, http://www.nytimes.com/2015/05/10/books/review/the-wright-brothers-by-david-mccullough.html.

32. Jeanne Clark, Joe Piccolo, Brian Stanton, and Karin Tyson, Patent Pools: A Solution to the Problem of Access in Biotechnology Patents? U.S. Patent and Trademark Office, December 5, 2000, http://www.uspto.gov/web/offices/pac/dapp/opla/patentpool.pdf, 4.

33. Manufacturers Aircraft Association v. U.S. 77 Ct. Cl. 481, 1933 WL 1818 (1933). The case cites government "insistence" that Wright and Curtiss joined the association.

34. Act of May 24, 1949, 81 Pub. L. No. 72, § 87, ch. 139. 63 Stat. 89, 102. 29 U.S.C. §1498 (2012).

35. James Love and Michael Palmedo, "Examples of Compulsory Licensing of Intellectual Property in the United States," CPTech background paper, September 29, 2001, http://www.cptech.org/ip/health/cl/us-cl.html, 1.

36. Ibid.; "KEI Research Note: Recent United States Compulsory Licenses," Knowledge Ecology International, March 7, 2014, http://keionline.org/sites/default/files/Annex_A_US_Compulsory_Licenses_7Mar2014_8_5x11.pdf, 1–2.

37. James Love, "Michael Froman's Decision in the Apple/Samsung ITC Patent Dispute and the USTR Trade Agenda," Knowledge Ecology International, August 5, 2013, http://keionline.org/node/1785.

38. Ellen t'Hoen, The Global Politics of Pharmaceutical Monopoly Power: Drug Patents, Access, Innovation and the Application of the WTO Doha Declaration on TRIPS and Public Health (Diemen, Netherlands: AMB, 2009), 43, http://www.msfaccess.org/sites/default/files/MSF_assets/Access/Docs/ACCESS_book_GlobalPolitics_tHoen_BNG_2009.pdf.

39. "KEI Research Note," 6.

40. "Compulsory Licensing. Chapter II: Government Use under 28 USC 1498," Knowledge Ecology International, http://www.cptech.org/ip/health/cl/us-1498.html.

41. James Love, "Open Letter to Those Who Collectively Produced the May 23, 2012 Statement to the WIPO SCP on the Topics of Patents and Health," Knowledge Ecology International, May 25, 2012, http://keionline.org/node/1420.

42. James Love, "Open Letter to Patent Office, on Its War against the Global Poor," Blog Huffington Post, May 25, 2012, http://www.huffingtonpost.com/james-love/open-letter-to-patentoff_b_1545232.html.

43. "KEI Research Note," 10.

44. Ylan Q. Mui, "President Trump Signs Order to Withdraw from Trans-Pacific Partnership," Washington Post, January 23, 2017, https://www.washingtonpost.com/news/wonk/wp/2017/01/23/president-trump-signs-order-to-withdraw-from-transpacific-partnership/?utm_term=.0c321ae17a15.

45. John Edwards, "What's Next after the US Withdrawal from the TPP?," Al Jazeera, http://www.aljazeera.com/indepth/opinion/2017/01/withdrawal-tpp-170126092759229.html, January 26, 2017.

46. "Text of the Trans-Pacific Partnership," New Zealand Foreign Affairs & Trade, Manatū Aorere, https://www.mfat.govt.nz/en/about-us/who-we-are/treaty-making-process/trans-pacific-partnership-tpp/text-of-the-trans-pacific-partnership (accessed June 17, 2016), art. 18.37.2 (evergreening), art. 18.53 (patent linkage), and art. 9.1(f) (ISDS). The TPP terms were kept secret from the public during years of negotiations, but it was hardly a surprise when they were revealed to be so favorable to pharmaceutical corporations. Big Pharma representatives were among the more than five hundred corporate advisers who were privy to the talks, but access-to-medicine advocates were shut out. Howard Schneider, "Trade Deals a Closely Held Secret, Shared by More than 500 Advisers," Washington Post, February 28, 2014, https://www.washingtonpost.com/business/economy/tradedeals-a-closely-held-secret-shared-bymore-than-500-advisers/2014/02/28/7daa65ec-9d99-11e3-a050-dc3322a94fa7_story.html.

47. Ellen R. Shaffer and Joseph E. Benner, "A Trade Agreement's Impact on Access to Generic Drugs," Health Affairs 28, no. 5 (2009): 957–68, doi: 10.1377/hlthaff.28.5.w957.

48. Rohit Malpani, "All Costs, No Benefits: How the US-Jordan Free Trade Agreement Affects Access to Medicines 206–17, Business Journal for the Generic Medicine Sector 6 (2009): 206–17, doi:10.1057/jgm.2009.13.

49. Dean Baker, "Prescription Drugs and the Trans-Pacific Partnership: Big Pharma Hit by Skills Shortage," Beat the Press, Center for Economic and Policy Research, March 26, 2016, http://cepr.net/blogs/beat-the-press/prescription-drugs-and-the-trans-pacific-partnership-big-pharma-hit-by-skills-shortage.

50. Hazel V. J. Moir, Brigitte Tenni, Deborah Gleeson, and Ruth Lopert, "The Trans-Pacific Partnership Agreement and Access to HIV Treatment in Vietnam," 1–14, Global Public Health (November 2016), http://www.pubpdf.com/pub/27841097/The-Trans-Pacific-Partnership-Agreement-and-access-to-HIV-treatment-in-Vietnam; Amy Kapczynski, Bhaven N. Sampat, and Kenneth C. Shadlen, "The TPP and Drug Prices: Not a Settled Matter," Foreign Affairs, October 28, 2016, https://www.foreignaffairs.com/articles/2016-10-28/tpp-and-drug-prices.

51. The U.S. Federal Trade Commission has concluded that the additional protection of data exclusivity is not a necessary addition to patent protection in the area of biologics. U.S. Federal Trade Commission, "Emerging Health Care Issues: Follow-On Biologic Drug Competition Federal Trade Commission Report," June 2009, vi–vii, https://www.ftc.gov/sites/default/files/documents/reports/emerging-health-care-issues-follow-biologic-drug-competition-federal-trade-commission-report/p083901biologicsreport.pdf. For a contrary view, see Kristina Lybecker, "The Sticking Point That Shouldn't Be: The Role of Pharmaceutical Patents in the TPP Negotiations," IPWatchdog, August 3, 2015, http://www.ipwatchdog.com/2015/08/03/role-of-pharmaceutical-patents-in-the-tpp-negotiations/id=60283/. Lybecker argues that data exclusivity is necessary for biologics because patent protection for biologics is narrower than with "small molecule" drugs: "[G]eneric drugs are required to contain the identical active ingredient. In contrast, in the production of biosimilars, effective variants are sufficient."

52. U.S. Food and Drug Administration, "What Are 'Biologics' Questions and Answers," http://www.fda.gov/AboutFDA/CentersOffices/OfficeofMedicalProductsandTobacco/CBER/ucm133077.htm (accessed June 16, 2016).

53. Christian Nordqvist, "One Year on Herceptin for Breast Cancer Ideal," Medical News Today, October 1, 2012, http://www.medicalnewstoday.com/articles/250912.php.

54. "Health Policy 101: How the Trans-Pacific Partnership Will Impact Prescription Drugs," Brookings Institution, May 19, 2015, https://www.brookings.edu/blog/health360/2015/05/19/health-policy-101-how-the-trans-pacific-partnership-will-impact-prescription-drugs/.

55. Trans-Pacific Partnership Agreement, art. 18.51

56. Ibid.

57. Spurred on by pharmaceutical corporations, the trade representative for the Obama administration argued hard for even longer terms of data exclusivity for TPP countries. Keith Bradsher and Andrew Pollack, "What Changes Lie Ahead from the Trans-Pacific Partnership Pact," New York Times, October 5, 2015, http://www.nytimes.com/2015/10/06/business/international/what-changes-lie-ahead-from-the-trans-pacific-partnership-pact.html. At least one prominent medicines advocate had said that the Obama administration has been "worse than the George W. Bush administration on these (access to medicines) issues." Network for Equitable Access to the Benefits of Research, "Obama Gets Thank You from Big Pharma at 2016 International AIDS Conference," press release, July 27, 2016, https://nearsrch.wordpress.com/2016/07/20/obama-gets-big-thank-you-from-big-pharma-at-2016-international-aids-conference/. Ironically, this position was taken even though the Obama administration itself had been pushing for a reduction in the United States to a data exclusivity term of seven years. That drop from the current national standard of twelve years would allow more purchases of cheaper biosimilars, saving over $4 billion in Medicare costs in just a decade. Dan Stanton, "Seven Year Market Exclusivity?" Biopharma Reporter, March 7, 2014, http://www.biopharma-reporter.com/Markets-Regulations/Seven-year-market-exclusivity-Industry-hits-out-at-Obama-s-pro-biosimilar-Budget; Ed Silverman,

"Bill Introduced to Speed Cheaper Versions of Pricey Biologics to Market," STAT, June 23, 2016, https://www.statnews.com/pharmalot/2016/06/23/congress-bill-biosimilar/?s_campaign=tw&utm_content=buffer0b2a4&utm_medium=social&utm_source=twitter.com&utm_campaign=buffer.

58. Union for Affordable Cancer Treatment, "UACT Letter to TPP Negotiators," July 26, 2015, http://cancerunion.org/files/UACT-TPP-26July2015.pdf. According to the letter, "It is important that the TPP, at a minimum, allows exceptions to rights in test data for cases when prices are excessive and/or a barrier to access, where there are shortages of drugs, when duplicative trials are unethical, or for other legitimate policy reasons. . . . Many cancer patients do not have time to waste." The negative impact of the TPP would not have been limited to poor countries: members of the U.S. Congress agreed that the TPP would have reduced the ability of the U.S. government to control medicine pricing in the future. Sam Baker, "Waxman Wants Biologic Drugs Kept out of Trade Talks," The Hill, August 4, 2011, http://thehill.com/policy/healthcare/175533-waxman-wants-biologic-drugs-kept-out-of-trade-talks.

59. Julia Belluz, "How the Trans-Pacific Partnership Could Drive Up the Cost of Medicine Worldwide," Vox, October 5, 2015, http://www.vox.com/2015/10/5/9454511/tpp-cost-medicine.

60. Ibid.

61. Zahara Heckscher, "TPP Threatens Access to Medicines," YubaNet, January 12, 2016, https://zaharaheckscher.com/2016/01/12/tpp-threatens-access-to-medicines-statement-in-advance-of-state-of-the-union/.

62. Joshua Meltzer, "The Significance of the Trans-Pacific Partnership for the United States," Brookings Institution, May 16, 2012, http://www.brookings.edu/research/testimony/2012/05/16-us-trade-strategy-meltzer.

19. Pharma-Pushed Trade Agreements Steal the Power of Democratically Elected Governments

1. Brook K. Baker and Katrina Geddes, "Corporate Power Unbound: Investor-State Arbitration of IP Monopolies on Medicines—Eli Lilly v. Canada and the Trans-Pacific Partnership Agreement," Research Papers Series No. 242–2015, Northeastern Public Law and Theory Faculty, September 29, 2015, http://papers.ssrn.com/sol3/papers.cfm?abstract_id=2667062.

2. Some advocates argue that ISDS provisions that suggest that the United States is liable for infringements on the intellectual property rights of foreign corporations violates a 1991 U.S. Supreme Court ruling, Fla. Prepaid Postsecondary Educ. Expense Bd. v. College Sav. Bank, 527 U.S. 627 (U.S. 1999), that suits against states for intellectual property infringements violates the Eleventh Amendment to the U.S. Constitution; Zack Struver and Tazio De Tomassi, "USTR Proposal in TPP Would Undermine State Sovereign Immunity for Patents, Copyrights, Expose U.S. Taxpayers to Fines under ISDS," Knowledge Ecology International, filmed July 26, 2015, 03:22 YouTube video, posted July 26, 2015, https://www.youtube.com/watch?v=RbVQZa85xVQ.

3. "Text of the Trans-Pacific Partnership," New Zealand Foreign Trade & Affairs: Manatū Aorere, https://www.mfat.govt.nz/en/about-us/who-we-are/treaty-making-process/trans-pacific-partnership-tpp/text-of-the-trans-pacific-partnership (accessed June 15, 2016). art. 9.1(f) (ISDS).

4. Yuki Noguchi, "Trans-Pacific Partnership Provision on Trade Disputes Draws Criticism," All Things Considered, National Public Radio, October 28, 2015, http://www.npr.org/2015/10/28/452608600/trans-pacific-partnership-provision-on-trade-disputes-draws-criticism?utm_source=npr_newsletter&utm_medium=email&utm_content=20151029&utm_campaign=npr_email_a_friend&utm_term=storyshare. Studies have shown that the inclusion of ISDS in trade agreements does not increase foreign direct investment, which is typically

the rationale provided to persuade governments to agree to those terms; Public Citizen, "As Growing European Government Opposition to Investor-State Regime Shadows This Week's U.S.-EU Talks, New Report Takes on Obama Administration Defense of Parallel Legal System for Foreign Corporations," news release, October 2, 2014, http://www.citizen.org/docu ments/press-release-isds-tafta-report-october-2014.pdf.

5. Harold Meyerson, "The Trade Clause That Overrules Governments," Washington Post, October 1, 2015, https://www.washingtonpost.com/opinions/harold-meyerson-allow ing-foreign-firms-to-sue-nations-hurts-trade-deals/2014/10/01/4b3725b0-4964-11e4-891d-713f052086a0_story.html; David Moberg, "8 Terrible Things about the Trans-Pacific Partnership," In These Times, December 16, 2015, http://inthesetimes.com/article/18695/TPP_ Free-Trade_Globalization_Obama.

6. Moberg, "8 Terrible Things."

7. Ante Wessels, "TPP: Rigged ISDS," Foundation for a Free Information Infrastructure (blog), November 5, 2015, https://blog.ffii.org/tpp-rigged-isds/.

8. Ibid.

9. Public Citizen, "As Growing European Government Opposition."

10. Ibid.

11. Don Lee, "Critics of Trans-Pacific Partnership Trade Deal Warn about Arbitration Clause," Los Angeles Times, August 19, 2015, http://www.latimes.com/business/la-fi-trade-court-dispute-20150819-story.html; Jim Armitage, "Big Tobacco Puts Countries on Trial as Concerns over TTIP Deals Mount," Independent, October 21, 2014, http://www.indepen dent.co.uk/news/business/analysis-and-features/big-tobacco-puts-countries-on-trial-as-con cerns-over-ttip-deals-mount-9807478.html.

12. Meyerson, "Trade Clause That Overrules Governments."

13. Yuki Noguchi, "Trans-Pacific Partnership Provision"; Public Citizen, "As Growing European Government Opposition"; "Ecuador's Highest Court vs. a Foreign Tribunal: Who Will Have the Final Say on Whether Chevron Must Pay a $9.5 Billion Judgment for Amazon Devastation?" Public Citizen, December 11 2013, http://citizen.typepad.com/eye sontrade/2013/12/ecuadors-highest-court-vs-a-foreign-tribunal-who-will-have-the-final-say-on-whether-chevron-will-pay.html.

14. Fran Quigley, "SDGs vs Trade Agreements: Not a Fair Fight," Health and Human Rights Journal, September 13, 2015, https://www.hhrjournal.org/2015/09/sdg-series-sus tainable-development-goals-vs-trade-agreements-not-a-fair-fight/. UN Secretary-General and Co-Chairs of the High-Level Panel, "Final Report: United Nations Secretary-General's High-Level Panel on Access to Health Technologies: Promoting Innovation and Access to Health Technologies," September 14, 2016, 33, http://www.unsgaccessmeds.org/final-report.

15. "U.S. Opponents of Trans-Pacific Partnership Say Keystone Suit Illustrates Threat from Trade Deal," Bloomberg News, January 7, 2016, http://calgaryherald.com/business/energy/u-s-opponents-of-trans-pacific-partnership-say-keystone-suit-illustrates-threat-from-trade-deal.

16. Joseph E. Stiglitz and Adam S. Hersh, "The Trans-Pacific Free-Trade Charade," Project Syndicate, October 2, 2015, https://www.project-syndicate.org/commentary/trans-pacific-partnership-charade-by-joseph-e--stiglitz-and-adam-s--hersh-2015-10#TvXkSb XMpKwUV2k4.99.

17. Health GAP, Global Access Project, "Trading Views: Real Debates on Key Issues in TPP," hearing on access to medicines—U.S. House of Representatives Ways and Means Committee Hearing, December 8, 2015, http://infojustice.org/wp-content/uploads/2015/12/ HGAP-Ways-Mean-Committee-Statement-TPP-and-Access-to-Medicines.final_.pdf; Ass'n for Molecular Pathology v. Myriad Genetics, Inc., 133 S. Ct. 2107 (U.S. 2013).

18. Eli Lilly and Company v. The Government of Canada, "Notice of Intent to Submit a Claim to Arbitration under NAFTA (13 June 2013) UNCT-14-2 (NAFTA/UNCITRAL)," http://www.italaw.com/sites/default/files/case-documents/italaw1530.pdf.

19. Brook Baker, "Threat of Pharmaceutical-Related IP Investment Rights in the Trans-Pacific Partnership Agreement: An Eli Lilly v. Canada Case Study," Investment Treaty News, International Institute for Sustainable Development, September 20, 2013, https://www.iisd.org/itn/2013/09/20/threat-of-pharmaceutical-related-ip-investment-rights-in-the-trans-pacific-partnership-agreement-an-eli-lilly-v-canada-case-study/.

20. James Love, "Despite Assurances to Contrary, Intellectual Property Covered Asset for TPP ISDS Mechanism," James Love's Blog, Knowledge Ecology International, November 5 2015, http://www.keionline.org/node/2358.

21. Meyerson, "Trade Clause That Overrules Governments." Public Citizen, "As Growing European Government Opposition."

22. Public Citizen, "As Growing European Government Opposition."

23. Nations Unies Droits de L'Homme: Huat-Cammissariat, "UN Experts Voice Concern over Adverse Impact of Free Trade and Investment Agreements on Human Rights," news release, June 2015, http://www.ohchr.org/FR/NewsEvents/Pages/DisplayNews.aspx?NewsID=16031&LangID=E#sthash.oeZiOTA1.dpuf.

24. Tariana Turia, Government of New Zealand, "Government Moves Forward with Plain Packaging of Tobacco Products," news release, February 19, 2013, https://www.Beehive.Govt.Nz/Release/Government-Moves-Forward-Plain-Packaging-Tobacco-Products; Stiglitz and Hersh, "Trans-Pacific Free-Trade Charade.

25. Noguchi, "Trans-Pacific Partnership Provision."

26. Ibid.; Wessels, "TPP"; Health GAP, Global Access Project, "Trading Views."

20. Current Law Provides Opportunities for Affordable Generic Medicines

1. Portions of this section were originally published as Fran Quigley, "Making Medicines Accessible: Alternatives to the Flawed Patent System," Health and Human Rights Journal, November 23, 2015, http://www.hhrjournal.org/2015/11/making-medicines-accessible-alternatives-to-the-flawed-patent-system-2/.

2. Quoted in Raymond A. Smith and Patricia D. Siplon, Drugs into Bodies: Global AIDS Treatment Activism (Westport, CT: Praeger, 2006), 57–58. The broad availability of compulsory licenses under current international intellectual property law was reaffirmed in 2016 by the U.N. High-Level Panel on Access to Medicines. UN Secretary-General and Co-Chairs of the High-Level Panel, "Final Report: United Nations Secretary-General's High-Level Panel on Access to Health Technologies: Promoting Innovation and Access to Health Technologies," September 14, 2016, 23, http://www.unsgaccessmeds.org/final-report.

3. World Trade Organization, "Ministerial Declaration of 14 November 2001" (Doha Declaration) WT/MIN(01)/DEC/1, 41 I.L.M. 746 (2002), paras. 4 and 5, https://www.wto.org/english/thewto_e/minist_e/min01_e/mindecl_trips_e.htm.

4. World Trade Organization, "Compulsory Licensing of Pharmaceuticals and TRIPS," last modified September, 2006, https://www.wto.org/english/tratop_e/trips_e/public_health_faq_e.htm.

5. World Trade Organization, "Ministerial Declaration of 14 November 2001," para. 7; Alex Lawson, "WTO Panel Inks 17-Year Drug Patent Waiver for Poor Nations," Law 360, November 6, 2015, http://www.law360.com/articles/724573/wto-panel-inks-17-year-drug-patent-waiver-for-poor-nations.

6. Ellen t'Hoen, The Global Politics of Pharmaceutical Monopoly Power: Drug Patents, Access, Innovation and the Application of the WTO Doha Declaration on TRIPS and Public Health (Diemen, Netherlands: AMB, 2009), http://www.msfaccess.org/sites/default/files/MSF_assets/Access/Docs/ACCESS_book_GlobalPolitics_tHoen_BNG_2009.pdf, 44–62.

7. Knowledge Ecology International, "Competition Commission (of South Africa) Concludes an Agreement with Pharmaceutical Firms," last modified December 10, 2003,

http://www.cptech.org/ip/health/sa/cc12102003.html; Vikas Bajaj and Andrew Pollack, " India Orders Bayer to License a Patented Drug," New York Times, March 12, 2012, http://www.nytimes.com/2012/03/13/business/global/india-overrules-bayer-allowing-generic-drug.html?_r=0.

8. Bajaj and Pollack, "India Orders Bayer."

9. Ellen t'Hoen, "Access to Cancer Treatment: A Study of Medicine Pricing Issues with Recommendations for Improving Access to Cancer Medication," Oxfam, February 2015, https://www.oxfam.org/sites/www.oxfam.org/files/file_attachments/rr-access-cancer-treatment-inequality-040215-en.pdf, 37.

10. Ibid., 38.

11. "Open Letter to Minister Davies Calling for Urgent Action to Adopt TRIPS Safeguards into Law," Fix the Patent Laws, October 29, 2015, http://www.fixthepatentlaws.org/?p=1034.

12. Bayh-Dole Act, Pub. L. No. 96-517, 94 Stat. 3015-28 (2000) (Bayh-Dole Act, 35 U.S.C. §§200–212 [2000 & Supp. II 2002]).

13. Ibid., sec. 202.

14. Alfred B. Engelberg and Aaron S. Kesselheim, "Use the Bayh-Dole Act to Lower Drug Prices for Government Healthcare Programs," Nature Medicine 22 (2016): 576, doi: 10.1038/nm0616-576.

15. Bhaven N. Sampat and Frank R. Lichtenberg, "What Are the Respective Roles of the Public and Private Sectors in Pharmaceutical Innovation?" Health Affairs 30, no. 2 (2011): 332–39, doi: 10.1377/hlthaff.2009.0917.

16. Ibid.

17. Office of Representative Lloyd Doggett, "Over 50 Members of Congress to Obama Administration: Help End Drug Price Gouging Now," news release, January 11, 2016, http://www.fiercepharma.com/press-releases/over-50-members-congress-obama-administration-help-end-drug-price-gouging-n.

18. Quoted in Ed Silverman, "NIH Asked to Fight Price Gouging by Overriding Drug Patents," Pharmalot, STAT, January 11, 2016, http://www.statnews.com/pharmalot/2016/01/11/nih-drug-costs-patents/.

19. Carolyn Y. Johnson, "Taxpayers Helped Fund This $129,000 Cancer Drug. Should the Government Help Cut the Price?" Wonkblog, Washington Post, January 14, 2016, https://www.washingtonpost.com/news/wonk/wp/2016/01/14/taxpayers-helped-fund-this-129000-cancer-drug-should-the-government-help-cut-the-price/.

20. Francis S. Collins, director of National Institutes of Health, letter to Andrew Goldman, Knowledge Ecology International, June 20, 2016, http://keionline.org/sites/default/files/Final-Response-Goldman-6.20.2016.pdf.

21. KEI WashDC, "Francis Collins and Senator Durbin on NIH March-In Rights, April 7, 2016, Senate Hearing," April, 2016, YouTube video, 4.22, September 2016, https://www.youtube.com/watch?v=wpo5sOQV9HY.

22. Ibid.; Peter S. Arno and Michael H. Davis, "Why Don't We Enforce Existing Drug Price Controls? The Unrecognized and Unenforced Reasonable Pricing Requirements Imposed upon Patents Deriving in Whole or in Part from Federally Funded Research," Tulane Law Review 75, no. 3 (2001):631–93. For an opposing view, see Birch Bayh and Robert Dole, "Our Law Helps Patients Get New Drugs Sooner," Washington Post, April 11, 2002, https://www.washingtonpost.com/archive/opinions/2002/04/11/our-law-helps-patients-get-new-drugs-sooner/d814d22a-6e63-4f06-8da3-d9698552fa24/. Bayh and Dole argue that price is not relevant to whether the government can issue generic licenses.

23. James Love, "Sanders Offers Amendment to Create Compulsory Licenses on Medical Inventions, for Veterans," James Love's Blog, Knowledge Ecology International, July 23, 2015, http://keionline.org/node/2290.

24. Amy Kapczynski and Aaron S. Kesselheim, "'Government Patent Use': A Legal Approach to Reducing Drug Spending," Health Affairs 35, no. 5, (2016): 791–97, doi: 10..1377/hlthaff.2015.1120; Zain Rizvi, Amy Kapczynski, and Aaron S. Kesselheim, "A Simple Way for the Government to Curb Inflated Drug Prices," Washington Post, May 12, 2016, https://www.washingtonpost.com/opinions/a-simple-way-for-the-government-to-curb-inflated-drug-prices/2016/05/12/ed89c9b4-16fc-11e6-aa55-670cabef46e0_story.html.

25. World Health Organization, "WHO Model List of Essential Medicines, 19th List," August 2015, http://www.who.int/selection_medicines/committees/expert/20/EML_2015_FINAL_amended_AUG2015.pdf?ua=1.

26. Sandeep Kishore, Kavitha Kolappa, Jordan D. Jarvis, Paul H. Park, Rachel Belt, Thirukumaran Balasubramaniam, and Rachel Kiddell-Monroe, "Overcoming Obstacles to Enable Access to Medicines for Noncommunicable Diseases in Poor Countries," Health Affairs 34, no. 9 (2015): 1569–77, doi: 10.1377/hlthaff.2015.0375.

27. Andy L. Gray, Veronika J. Wirtz, Ellen F. M. t'Hoen, Michael R. Reich, and Hans V. Hogerzeil, "Essential Medicines Are Still Essential," Lancet 368 (2015): 1601–3, doi: http://dx.doi.org/10.1016/S01406736(15)60460-3.

28. Kishore et al., "Overcoming Obstacles." One of the positive effects of adding key new medicines to the Essential Medicines List was to blunt the argument from some pharmaceutical industry spokespersons that patent protection is not a barrier to medicines access because the previous list contained few medicines under patent. See, Andrew Witty, "Scaling Up for Universal Health Coverage," The Lancet, November 7, 2016, http://yolse.org/wp-content/uploads/2016/11/EssentialMeds.pdf, 7. The updated list includes a dozen medicines whose availability is compromised by monopoly patent protection. Ellen t'Hoen, Private Patents and Public Health: Changing Intellectual Property Rules for Access to Medicines (Health Action International, 2016), http://accesstomedicines.org/wp-content/uploads/private-patents-and-public-health.pdf, 101.

29. World Health Organization, "WHO Moves to Improve Access To Lifesaving Medicines for Hepatitis C, Drug-Resistant TB and Cancers, "news release, May 8, 2015, http://www.who.int/mediacentre/news/releases/2015/new-essential-medicines-list/en/.

30. Kishore et al., "Overcoming Obstacles"; Stop TB Partnership, "What Is the GDF?" http://stoptb.org/gdf/whatis/default.asp (accessed June 16, 2016).

31. Medicines Patent Pool, Working Today for the Treatments of Tomorrow: Annual Report 2014, http://www.medicinespatentpool.org/wp-content/uploads/MPP_Annual_Report_2014_web.pdf; GlaxoSmithKline, "GSK Expands Graduated Approach to Patents and Intellectual Property to Widen Access to Medicines in the World's Poorest Countries," news release, March 31, 2016, http://www.gsk.com/en-gb/media/press-releases/2016/gsk-expands-graduated-approach-to-patents-and-intellectual-property-to-widen-access-to-medicines-in-the-world-s-poorest-countries/.

32. Veronika J. Wirtz, Hans V. Hogerzeil, Andrew L. Gray, Maryam Bigdeli, Cornelis P. de Joncheere, Margaret A. Ewen, Martha Gyansa-Lutterodt, Sun Jing, Vera L. Luiza, Regina M Mbindyo, Helene Möller, Corrina Moucheraud, Bernard Pécoul, Lembit Rägo, Arash Rashidian, Dennis Ross-Degnan, Peter N. Stephens, Yot Teerawattananon, Ellen F. M. 't Hoen, Anita K Wagner, Prashant Yadav, Michael R. Reich, "Essential Medicines for Universal Health Coverage," The Lancet, November 7, 2016, http://yolse.org/wp-content/uploads/2016/11/EssentialMeds.pdf, 65.

33. Aaron Cosbey, "Brave New Deal? Assessing the May 10th U.S. Bipartisan Compact on Free Trade Agreements," Institute for Sustainable Democracy, August 2007, https://www.iisd.org/pdf/2007/com_brave_new_deal.pdf.

34. Médecins Sans Frontières/Doctors Without Borders, "Open Letter to ASEAN Governments: Don't Trade Away Health," last modified February 4, 2016, https://www.msfaccess.org/content/msf-open-letter-asean-governments-dont-trade-away-health; Representative Sander Levin, "Why I Oppose TPP," Medium, February 18, 2016, medium.com/@repsandylevin/why-i-oppose-tpp-1810dec2a79d#.z1kdkmvgn.

35. World Trade Organization, "Agreement on Trade-Related Aspects of Intellectual Property Rights (TRIPS)," art. 27, April 15, 1994, https://www.wto.org/english/tratop_e/trips_e/t_agm0_e.htm.

36. Marcus Low and Eduard Grebe, "Transnational Mobilisation on Access to Medicines: The Global Movement around the Imatinib Mesylate Case and Its Roots in the AIDS Movement," December 31, 2014, doi: http://dx.doi.org/10.2139/ssrn.2546392. Also, in the United States, private organizations are now making concerted efforts to challenge the legitimacy of over a dozen drug patents; Gretchen Morgenson, "Working to Lower Drug Costs by Challenging Questionable Patents," New York Times, November 27, 2015, http://www.nytimes.com/2015/11/29/business/working-to-lower-drug-costs-by-challenging-questionable-patents.html?action=click&pgtype=Homepage&clickSource=story-heading&module=second-column-region&region=top-news&WT.nav=top-news.

37. "A Question of Utility: Patents Are Protected by Governments Because They Are Held to Promote Innovation. But There Is Plenty of Evidence That They Do Not," Economist, August 8, 2015, http://www.economist.com/node/21660559?zid=317&ah=8a47fc455a44945580198768fad0fa41. The article notes that no pending U.S. congressional proposal seeks abolition patents because "any lawmaker brave enough to propose doing away with them altogether, or raising similar questions about the much longer monopolies given to copyright holders, would face an onslaught from the intellectual-property lobby." See also, in reference to U.S. lobbying and campaign contribution investments by the pharmaceutical industry, Statista, "Top Lobbying Industries in the United States in 2014," http://www.statista.com/statistics/257364/top-lobbying-industries-in-the-us/ (accessed June 16, 2016); "Top Interest Groups Giving to Members of Congress, 2016 Cycle," OpenSecrets.org, http://www.opensecrets.org/industries/mems.php (accessed June 15, 2016).

38. Marc-André Gagnon and Sidney Wolfe, Mirror, Mirror on the Wall: Medicare Part D Pays Needlessly High Brand-Name Drug Prices Compared with Other OECD Countries and with U.S. Government Programs (Washington, DC: Carleton University and Public Citizen, 2015), http://freepdfhosting.com/ff84833f9f.pdf, 7.

39. German Lopez, "After Public Outcry, Pharmaceutical Company to Cut Price of Drug It Hiked by 5,500 Percent" Vox, September 22, 2015, http://www.vox.com/2015/9/22/9375295/turing-daraprim-price-cut.

40. Ibid.

41. Quoted in Dan Goldberg, "Cuomo Enters National Debate with Proposal to Cap Drug Prices," Politico New York, January 20, 2016, http://www.capitalnewyork.com/article/albany/2016/01/8588431/cuomo-enters-national-debate-proposal-cap-drug-prices; Dylan Scott, "Big Pharma's Big Question: Is Trump Friend or Foe?" STAT, November 9, 2016, https://www.statnews.com/2016/11/09/trump-drug-prices/.

42. Jonathan D. Rockoff, "Rising Drug Costs to Be in Focus at Congressional Heating," Wall Street Journal, December 5, 2015, http://www.wsj.com/articles/rising-drug-costs-to-be-in-focus-at-congressional-hearing-1449311407.

43. Jill Wechsler, "Politics and Pricing Will Challenge Manufacturers in 2016," Pharmaceutical Technology 40, no. 1 (2016): 26–29, http://www.pharmtech.com/politics-and-pricing-will-challenge-manufacturers-2016.

44. Ibid.

45. Social Security Act, 42 U.S.C. 1395w-111 (2016); Pub L. 108–73, § 1860D-11 (2016).

46. Gagnon and Wolfe, Mirror, Mirror on the Wall.

47. The pharmaceutical industry also uses its financial power to exert significant influence over the critical drug-approval process by the FDA, by providing operating funds to the agency, contributing financially to the experts who form the FDA advisory committees on drug approvals, and exerting political pressure on key agency appointments; Marcia Angell, The Truth about the Drug Companies: How They Deceive Us and What to Do about It (New York: Random House, 2004), 208–14.

48. Barack Obama, "United States Health Care Reform: Progress to Date and Next Steps," Journal of the American Medical Association 316, no. 5 (2016): 525–32, doi: 10.1001/jama.2016.9797.

49. Nadia Kounang, "Why Pharmaceuticals Are Cheaper Abroad," CNN, September 28, 2015, http://www.cnn.com/2015/09/28/health/us-pays-more-for-drugs/.

50. Ashley Kirzinger, Bryan Wu, and Mollyann Brodie, "Kaiser Health Tracking Poll: September 2016," Kaiser Family Foundation, last modified September 29, 2016, http://kff.org/report-section/kaiser-health-tracking-poll-september-2016-politics-and-rx-costs/.

51. Peter Sullivan, "Trump Calls for Medicare to Negotiate Drug Prices," The Hill, January 26, 2016, http://thehill.com/policy/healthcare/267005-trump-calls-for-medicare-to-nego tiate-drug-prices; Laura Lorenzetti, "Hillary Clinton Releases Health Plan That Aims to Combat Skyrocketing Drug Costs," Fortune, September 22, 2015, http://fortune.com/2015/09/22/hillary-clinton-drug-price-plan/.

52. Quoted in Steven Ross Johnson, " CEO Power Panel: Healthcare Leaders Back Feds Stepping in to Restrain Drug Prices," ModernHealthcare.com, November 14, 2015, http://www.modernhealthcare.com/article/20151114/MAGAZINE/311149963.

53. PHARMAC, "How Medicines Are Funded," last modified January 16, 2016, http://www.pharmac.govt.nz/medicines/how-medicines-are-funded/.

54. For a discussion of how such negotiation would work in the United States, see Topher Spiro, Maura Calsyn, and Thomas Huelskoetter, "Negotiation Plus: A Framework for Value-Based Drug Pricing Negotiation," Center for American Progress, September 26, 2016, https://www.americanprogress.org/issues/healthcare/reports/2016/09/26/144760/nego tiation-plus-a-framework-for-value-based-drug-pricing-negotiation/.

55. Paul T. Menzel, "Are Patents an Efficient and Internationally Fair Means of Funding Research and Development for New Medicines?" in Ethics and the Business of Biomedicine, ed. Denis G. Arnold, 62–82 (Cambridge, UK: Cambridge University Press, 2009).

56. Knowledge Ecology International, "2015–2016 Pharmaceutical Transparency Legislation," http://keionline.org/sites/default/files/transparency-legislation-summary-kei-briefing-note-2016-2.pdf.

57. Donald Light and Rebecca Warburton, "Demythologizing the High Costs of Pharmaceutical Research," BioSocieties 6, no. 1 (2011): 1–17, http://www.pharmamyths.net/files/Bio societies_2011_Myths_of_High_Drug_Research_Costs.pdf.

58. Andrew Pollack, "Drug Prices Soar, Prompting Calls for Justification," New York Times, July 23, 2015, http://www.nytimes.com/2015/07/23/business/drug-companies-pushed-from-far-and-wide-to-explain-high-prices.html; Robert Weisman, "Bill to Rein in Drug Costs Spurs Controversy," Boston Globe, April 11, 2016, https://www.bostonglobe.com/busi ness/2016/04/11/drug-price-control-bill-gets-mass-hearing/Brd6HGfbhIUDFvnFxpMxaP/story.html. Ed Silverman, "California Senator Introduces a New Bill For Transparency in Drug Pricing," STAT, December 6, 2016, https://www.statnews.com/pharmalot/2016/12/06/california-drug-prices-transparency-2/.

59. "Editorial: Bill on Drug Pricing Would Help State on Figuring Healthcare Costs," Los Angeles Times, April 26, 2015, http://www.latimes.com/opinion/editorials/la-ed-drug-prices-transparency-20150426-story.html.

60. Parliamentary Assembly, Council of Europe, "Measures to Encourage Drug Companies to Respond Better to Public Health Needs," September 29, 2015, http://www.assembly.coe.int/nw/xml/News/News-View-EN.asp?newsid=5794&lang=2&cat=8.

61. Laura Lorenzetti, "Hillary Clinton"; Gregg Gonsalves, "Martin Shkreli Is Just a Tiny Part of a Huge Problem," Nation, September 25, 2015, http://www.thenation.com/article/martin-shkreli-is-just-a-tiny-part-of-a-huge-problem/; Dean Baker, Rigged: How Globalization and the Rules of the Modern Economy Were Structured to Make the Rich Richer (Washington, DC: Center for Economic and Policy Research, 2016), 103–105. Gonsalves and Baker both suggest shortening patent terms. Ayalew Tefferi, Hagop Kantarjian, S. Vincent Rajkumar, Lawrence H. Baker, Jan L. Abkowitz, John W. Adamson, Ranjana Hira Advani, James Allison, Karen H. Antman, Robert C. Bast Jr., John M. Bennett, Edward J. Benz Jr., Nancy Berliner, Joseph Bertino, Ravi Bhatia, Smita Bhatia, Deepa Bhojwani, Charles D. Blanke, Clara D. Bloomfield, Linda Bosserman, Hal E. Broxmeyer, John C. Byrd, Fernando Cabanillas, George Peter Canellos, Bruce A. Chabner, Asher Chanan-Khan, Bruce Cheson, Bayard Clarkson, Susan L. Cohn, Gerardo Colon-Otero, Jorge Cortes, Steven Coutre, Massimo Cristofanilli, Walter J. Curran Jr., George Q. Daley, Daniel J. DeAngelo, H. Joachim Deeg, Lawrence H. Einhorn, Harry P. Erba, Francisco J. Esteva, Elihu Estey, Isaiah J. Fidler, James Foran, Stephen Forman, Emil Freireich, Charles Fuchs, James N. George, Morie A. Gertz, Sergio Giralt, Harvey Golomb, Peter Greenberg, Jordan Gutterman, Robert I. Handin, Samuel Hellman, Paulo Marcelo Hoff, Ronald Hoffman, Waun Ki Hong, Mary Horowitz, Gabriel N. Hortobagyi, Clifford Hudis, Jean Pierre Issa, Bruce Evan Johnson, Philip W. Kantoff, Kenneth Kaushansky, David Khayat, Fadlo R. Khuri, Thomas J. Kipps, Margaret Kripke, Robert A. Kyle, Richard A. Larson, Theodore S. Lawrence, Ross Levine, Michael P. Link, Scott M. Lippman, Sagar Lonial, Gary H. Lyman, Maurie Markman, John Mendelsohn, Neal J. Meropol, Yoav Messinger, Therese M. Mulvey, Susan O'Brien, Roman Perez-Soler, Raphael Pollock, Josef Prchal, Oliver Press, Jerald Radich, Kanti Rai, Saul A. Rosenberg, Jacob M. Rowe, Hope Rugo, Carolyn D. Runowicz, Brenda M. Sandmaier, Alan Saven, Andrew I. Schafer, Charles Schiffer, Mikkael A. Sekeres, Richard T. Silver, Lillian L. Siu, David P. Steensma, F. Marc Stewart, Wendy Stock, Richard Stone, Rainer Storb, Louise C. Strong, Martin S. Tallman, Michael Thompson, Naoto T. Ueno, Richard A. Van Etten, Julie M. Vose, Peter H. Wiernik, Eric P. Winer, Anas Younes, Andrew D. Zelenetz, and Charles A. LeMaistre, "In Support of a Patient-Driven Initiative and Petition to Lower the High Cost of Cancer Drugs," Mayo Clinic Proceedings 90, no. 8 (2015): 996–1000, http://www.mayoclinicproceedings.org/article/S0025-6196(15)00430-9/pdf; Ed Silverman, "With Trump in Office, Senators Again Urge Importing Meds From Canada to Fight High Prices," STAT, February 14, 2017, https://www.statnews.com/pharmalot/2017/02/14/trump-canada-drug-prices-marathon/ (cancer physicians and U.S. Senators supporting importation of medicines from Canada); National Academy for State Health Policy, "States and the Rising Cost of Pharmaceuticals: A Call to Action," http://nashp.org/wp-content/uploads/2016/10/Rx-Paper.pdf, 7–8. The National Academy for State Health Policy proposes that pharma companies be treated as utilities. Alfred Engelberg, "Memo to the President: The Pharmaceutical Monopoly Adjustment Act of 2017," Health Affairs Blog, September 13, 2016, http://healthaffairs.org/blog/2016/09/13/memo-to-the-president-the-pharmaceutical-monopoly-adjustment-act-of-2017/. Engelberg addresses anti-evergreening proposals.

62. "Physicians Call for Fairness in Drug Prices, Availability," AMA Wire, November 17, 2015, http://www.ama-assn.org/ama/ama-wire/post/physicians-call-fairness-drug-prices-availability?utm_source=FBPAGE&utm_medium=Social_AMA&utm_term=281158990&utm_content=other&utm_campaign=article_alert.

63. "Proposals for Change: Transparency, Competition and Value," blog, Campaign for Sustainable Rx Pricing, April 25, 2016, http://www.csrxp.org/proposals-for-change-transparency-competition-and-value/.

21. There Is a Better Way to Develop Medicines

1. Alexandra Greenberg and Rachel Kiddell-Monroe, "ReRouting Biomedical Innovation: Observations From a Mapping of the Alternative Research and Development (R&D) Landscape," Global Health, September 24, 2016, https://www.ncbi.nlm.nih.gov/pmc/articles/PMC5024495/.

2. National Institutes of Health, "Budget," April 4, 2016, https://www.nih.gov/about-nih/what-we-do/budget;. Samuel Broder, "The Development of Antiretroviral Therapy and Its Impact on the HIV-1/AIDS Pandemic," Antiviral Research 85, no. 1 (2010), doi: 10.1016/j.antiviral.2009.10.002; National Institutes of Health, "Nobel Laureates," October 28, 2015, http://www.nih.gov/about-nih/what-we-do/nih-almanac/nobel-laureates.

3. Amy Maxmen, "Busting the Billion-Dollar Myth: How to Slash the Cost of Drug Development," Nature, August 24, 2016, http://www.nature.com/news/busting-the-billion-dollar-myth-how-to-slash-the-cost-of-drug-development-1.20469#auth-1.

4. Drugs for Neglected Diseases Initiative, "About Us," http://www.dndi.org/about-us/overview-dndi.html (accessed November 6, 2016).

5. Ellen t'Hoen, "Access to Cancer Treatment: A Study of Medicine Pricing Issues with Recommendations for Improving Access to Cancer Medication," Oxfam, February 2015, https://www.oxfam.org/sites/www.oxfam.org/files/file_attachments/rr-access-cancer-treatment-inequality-040215-en.pdf, 8, 42. Donald Light and Antonio Maturo, Good Pharma: The Public-Health Model of the Mario Negri Institute (Palgrave Macmillan 2015

6. Michael Kremer and Rachel Glennerster, Strong Medicine, Creating Incentives for Pharmaceutical Research and Neglected Diseases (Princeton: Princeton University Press, 2004).

7. Els Torreele and Piero Olliaro, "Why Ebola Should Be a Wake-Up Call for Drug Development," Voices, Open Society Foundations, November 21, 2014, https://www.opensocietyfoundations.org/voices/why-ebola-should-be-wake-call-drug-development.

8. James Love, "Annotated Bibliography of Articles and Books on Innovation Prizes," Knowledge Ecology International, 2012, http://keionline.org/prizes/cites; Joseph Stiglitz. "Scrooge and Intellectual Property Rights: A Medical Prize Fund Could Improve the Financing of Drug Innovations," British Medical Journal 333 (2006):1279–80, doi: http://academiccommons.columbia.edu/catalog/ac:148182.

9. Vijay Goel, "Charles Lindbergh and the Orteig Prize," Innovation in the Crowd, March 1, 2011, http://www.innovationinthecrowd.com/2011/03/01/charles-lindbergh-and-the-orteig-prize/.

10. James Love and Tim Hubbard, "Prizes for Innovation of New Medicines and Vaccines," Annals of Health Law 18, no. 2 (2009): 155–86, http://lawecommons.luc.edu/cgi/viewcontent.cgi?article=1111&context=annals.

11. Mat Todd, "In Drug Development, Openness Can Compete with Secrecy, Given the Chance," PLoS Blogs, October 22, 2015, http://blogs.plos.org/yoursay/2015/10/22/talking-drug-prices-pt-6-openness-vs-secrecy-in-drug-development-by-mat-todd/.

12. Health Impact Fund, "What Is Health Impact Fund?" http://healthimpactfund.org/#firstPage (accessed June 16, 2016).

13. European Commission, "German Company Wins EU's €2 Million Inducement Prize for Innovative Vaccine Technology," news release, March 10, 2014, http://europa.eu/rapid/press-release_IP-14-229_bn.htm; NHS England, "NHS Innovation Challenge Prizes," https://www.england.nhs.uk/challengeprizes/; Nesta, "Longitude Prize Open" https://longitudeprize.org/ (accessed June 16, 2016). Because vaccines and antibiotics are usually administered for

limited periods of time, some for-profit companies do not see them as particularly promising revenue producers once they are developed; Akshat Rathi, "To Fight Antibiotic Resistance, We May Have to Pay the Hugely Profitable Pharma Industry Even More," Quartz, May 20, 2015, http://qz.com/406959/to-fight-antibiotic-resistance-we-may-have-to-pay-the-hugely-profitable-pharma-industry-even-more/.

14. "A Question of Utility: Patents Are Protected by Governments Because They Are Held to Promote Innovation. But There Is Plenty of Evidence That They Do Not," Economist August 8, 2015, http://www.economist.com/node/21660559?zid=317&ah=8a47fc455a4494 5580198768fad0fa41.

15. Ernst Berndt, Rachel Glennerster, Jean Lee, Ruth Levine, Georg Weizsäcker, and Heidi Williams, "Advance Market Commitments for Vaccines against Neglected Diseases: Estimating Costs and Effectiveness," Health Economics 16, no. 5 (2007): 491–511, doi: 10.1002/hec.1176.

16. Ashley J. Stevens, Jonathan J. Jensen, Katrine Wyller, Patrick C. Kilgore, Sabarni Chatterjee, and Mark L. Rohrbaugh, "The Role of Public-Sector Research in the Discovery of Drugs and Vaccines," New England Journal of Medicine 364 (2011): 535–41, doi: 10.1056/ NEJMsa1008268; Bhaven Sampat and Frank Lichtenberg, "What Are the Respective Roles of the Public and Private Sectors in Pharmaceutical Innovation?" Health Affairs 30, no. 2 (2011): 332–39, doi: 10.1377/hlthaff.2009.0917; Jordan Rau, "Medicare Reveals How Much It Spends on Prescription Drugs for Americans," PBS Newshour, May 1, 2015, http://www. pbs.org/newshour/rundown/medicare-reveals-much-spends-prescription-drugs-americans/.

17. Dean Baker, Financing Drug Research: What Are the Issues? (Washington, DC: Center for Economic and Policy Research, 2004), http://cepr.net/documents/publications/intellec tual_property_2004_09.pdf.

18. Richard Anderson, "Pharmaceutical Industry Gets High on Fat Profits," BBC News, November 6, 2014, http://www.bbc.com/news/business-28212223.

19. Meredith Cohn, " Industry Funds Six Times More Clinical Trials Than Feds, Research Shows," Baltimore Sun, December 15, 2015, http://www.baltimoresun.com/health/bs-hs-trial-funding-20151214-story.html.

20. Médicins Sans Frontières/Doctors Without Borders, "Access Campaign: The 3P Project," MSF Access Campaign, last modified February 3, 2014, http://www.msfaccess.org/ sites/default/files/TB%20demo%20project%20extended%20version%20For%20 Web_12032014.pdf.

21. Aarthi Rao, Can a R&D Tax Credit Expand Investment in Product Development for Global Health? (Washington, DC: Results for Development Institute, February 28, 2011), http://healthresearchpolicy.org/sites/healthresearchpolicy.org/files/assessments/files/Tax%20 Credit%20Draft%20Consultation%20Draft%202%2028.pdf, 10–11. The Orphan Drug Act has been so successful in inducing innovation that some critics contend its incentives have been exploited by the pharmaceutical industry; Ken Armstrong and Michael Berens, "Pharma's Windfall: The Mining of Rare Diseases," Seattle Times, November 11, 2013, http://apps. seattletimes.com/reports/pharma-windfall/2013/nov/9/mining-rare-diseases/; Dina Gusovky, "How a Blockbuster Drug Can Become a Subsidized 'Orphan', CNBC Explains," CNBC, December 2, 2015, http://www.cnbc.com/2015/12/01/an-obscure-fda-rule-adding-to-drug-company-profits.html.

22. Orphanet, "About Orphan Drugs," last modified October 10, 2013, http://www. orpha.net/national/AU-EN/index/about-orphan-drugs/.

23. Portions of this section were originally published as Fran Quigley, "A Bitter Pill: Can Access to Medicine Advocates Score Another Victory?" Foreign Affairs, October 18, 2015, https://www.foreignaffairs.com/articles/south-africa/2015-10-18/bitter-pill.

24. An excellent profile of James Love is found in Sarah Bosely, "Big Pharma's Worst Nightmare," Guardian, January 26, 2016, http://www.theguardian.com/society/2016/jan/26/big-pharmas-worst-nightmare.

25. James Love, telephone interview with the author, September 15, 2015.

26. Ibid.

27. James Love and Tim Hubbard, "The Big Idea: Prizes to Stimulate R&D for New Medicines," Chicago-Kent Law Review, 82 (2007): 1520–54, http://studentorgs.kentlaw.iit.edu/cklawreview/wp-content/uploads/sites/3/vol82no3/Love.pdf; U.S. Senate, Committee on Health, Education, Labor and Pensions, S.R. 627—The Medical Innovation Prize Fund Act, 113th Congress, 2013, https://www.congress.gov/bill/113th-congress/senate-bill/627.

28. Ibid.

29. Suzanne Hill and Marie Paule Kieny, "Towards Access 2030," The Lancet, November 7, 2016, http://yolse.org/wp-content/uploads/2016/11/EssentialMeds.pdf, 5-6.

30. Dean Baker, Rigged: How Globalization and the Rules of the Modern Economy Were Structured to Make the Rich Richer (Washington, DC: Center for Economic and Policy Research, 2016), 103–105.

31. Love is not the only one who argues for delinkage. For example, Adam Mannan and Alan Story, writing in the 2006 anthology Power of Pills, made the moral case for eliminating the product patent for medicines. "Succinctly, the patent is the wrong incentive in the wrong direction; obtaining and distributing cures to diseases ought to come before pecuniary profit. In a civilized world ought we or should we let people die so that the pharmaceutical industry can charge the rest of us a few more dollars for a few more years on their 600 per cent mark-up? The principal bars to medicine access are not found in a deficit of manufacturing capacity or the lack of distribution infrastructure; rather they subsist in high drug prices or a dearth of medicine development. At the root of this barrier lies the patent system. . . . Abolish the product patent: it is pernicious to world health. Medicines were invented long before the product patent existed and abolishing it will save billions of lives." Adam Mannan and Alan Story, "Abolishing the Product Patent: A Step Forward for Global Access to Drugs," in Power of Pills: Social, Ethical and Legal Issues in Drug Development, Marketing and Pricing, ed. Jillian Clare Cohen, Patricia Illingworth and Udo Schüklenk (Ann Arbor, MI: Pluto Press, 2006), 181.

32. "Question of Utility."

33. World Health Organization (WHO), World Intellectual Property Organization (WIPO), and World Trade Organization (WTO), "Promoting Access to Medical Technologies and Innovation. Intersections between Public Health, Intellectual Property and Trade," February 5, 2013, 116–19, http://www.who.int/phi/promoting_access_medical_innovation/en/. Veronika J. Wirtz, Hans V. Hogerzeil, Andrew L. Gray, Maryam Bigdeli, Cornelis P. de Joncheere, Margaret A. Ewen, Martha Gyansa-Lutterodt, Sun Jing, Vera L Luiza, Regina M Mbindyo, Helene Möller, Corrina Moucheraud, Bernard Pécoul, Lembit Rägo, Arash Rashidian, Dennis Ross-Degnan, Peter N. Stephens, Yot Teerawattananon, Ellen F. M. 't Hoen, Anita K Wagner, Prashant Yadav, Michael R. Reich, "Essential Medicines for Universal Health Coverage," The Lancet, November 7, 2016, http://yolse.org/wp-content/uploads/2016/11/EssentialMeds.pdf, 64.

34. Ibid.

35. Fran Quigley, "The Sustainable Development Goals vs. Trade Agreements: Not a Fair Fight," Health and Human Rights Journal (blog), September 14, 2015, http://www.hhrjournal.org/2015/09/sdg-series-sustainable-development-goals-vs-trade-agreements-not-a-fair-fight/.

36. United Nations Secretary-General's High-Level Panel on Access to Medicines, "The Panel," http://www.unsgaccessmeds.org/new-page/ (accessed June 16, 2016).

37. Stephen Lewis, telephone interview with the author, December 15, 2015.

38. UN Secretary-General and Co-Chairs of the High-Level Panel, "Final Report: United Nations Secretary-General's High-Level Panel on Access to Health Technologies: Promoting Innovation and Access to Health Technologies," September 14, 2016, 12, http://www.unsgac cessmeds.org/final-report.

39. Ibid., 16, 29.

40. Ibid., 61.

41. Ibid., 10; Fran Quigley, "UN Report Adds to Momentum for Medicines Reform," Health and Human Rights Journal (blog) September 25, 2016, https://www.hhrjournal. org/2016/09/un-report-adds-to-momentum-for-medicines-reform/.

42. World Health Organization, "Research and Development to Meet Health Needs in Developing Countries: Strengthening Global Financing and Coordination. Report of the Consultative Expert Working Group on Research and Development: Financing and Coordination," 110–11, http://www.who.int/phi/cewg_report/en/; Surie Moon and Ellen t'Hoen, "Medicines for the World: A Global R&D Treaty Could Boost Innovation and Improve the Health of the World's Poor—and Rich," Scientist, October 1, 2012, http://www.thescientist. com/?articles.view/articleNo/32664/title/Medicines-for-the-World/.

43. Ryan Abbott, "Inside Views: Potential Elements of the WHO Global R&D Treaty: Tailoring Solutions for Disparate Contexts," Intellectual Property Watch, January 29, 2013, http://www.ip-watch.org/2013/01/29/potential-elements-of-the-who-global-rd-treaty-tailoring-solutions-for-disparate-contexts/.

44. Universities Allied for Essential Medicines, "About Us," http://uaem.org/who-we-are/ (accessed June 17, 2016).

45. Quoted in William New, "University Students Energise Global Campaign for Medical R&D Agreement," Intellectual Property Watch, May 1, 2016, http://www.ip-watch. org/2016/01/05/university-students-energise-global-campaign-for-medical-rd-agreement/.

46. Universities Allied for Essential Medicines, "Make Medicines for People, Not Profit," last modified November, 2015, https://uaem.wufoo.com/forms/make-medicines-for-people-not-for-profit/.

47. Ibid.

48. "Essential Medicines for Universal Health Coverage," The Lancet, November 7, 2016, http://yolse.org/wp-content/uploads/2016/11/EssentialMeds.pdf, 64-65.

49. Thiru Balasubramaniam, "WHA69: Resolution WHA69.23 on CEWG Follow-Up Charts Course for WHO's Work on R&D," Thiru's Blog, Knowledge Ecology International, May 28, 2016, http://keionline.org/node/2582.

22. Human Rights Law Demands Access to Essential Medicines

1. Portions of this section were originally published as Fran Quigley, "For Goodness' Sake: A Two-Part Proposal for Remedying the U.S. Charity/Justice Imbalance," Virginia Journal of Social Policy and Law 23, no. 1 (2016): 39–88, http://www.vjspl.org/wp-content/ uploads/2016/03/2-Articles-Quigley_Proposal-for-Remedying-Charity-Justice-Imbalance_ WD_1.26.pdf.

2. For examples, see Amos 5:24; Isaiah 58:6; Luke 4:16–18; Matthew 25: 39–45.

3. For example, Qur'an 16:90: "Indeed, Allah orders justice and good conduct and giving to relatives and forbids immorality and bad conduct and oppression." For Confucianism, Joseph Chan, "Making Sense of Confucian Justice," Polylog: Forum for Intercultural Philosophy, last modified 2001, http://them.polylog.org/3/fcj-en.htm: "A just society therefore has the following features: 1) Sufficiency for all —there is state provision to ensure that each citizen enjoys a level of material goods sufficient to live a good life. First priority would be given

to the poor and needy" (3). See also Mary Ann Glendon, A World Made New: Eleanor Roosevelt and the Universal Declaration of Human Rights (New York: Random House, 2002); Glendon quotes Peng-chun Chang's 1946 speech to the Economic and Social Council in support of economic and social rights: "Provisions are made for the aged, employment is provided for the able-bodied and education is afforded to the young. Widows and widowers, orphans and the childless, the deformed and the diseased, all are cared for" (185).

4. "Augustine of Hippo Quotes," The European Graduate School, http://www.egs.edu/library/augustine-of-hippo/quotes/ (accessed June 17, 2016).

5. Glendon, World Made New, 185–86. Glendon cites provisions in the eighteenth-century Prussian General Code, the nineteenth-century Norwegian Constitution, multiple French constitutions, the social insurance programs of late-nineteenth-century Germany, and the U.S. poor relief systems from the same era.

6. Ibid. See also David P. Currie, "Positive and Negative Constitutional Rights," University of Chicago Law Review 53 (1986): 865.

7. For example, Convention Limiting the Hours of Work in Industrial Undertakings to Eight in the Day and Forty-Eight in the Week (adopted November 28, 1919, entered into force June 13, 1921), Convention Concerning Minimum Standards of Social Security (adopted June 28, 1952, 210 U.N.T.S. 131, entered into force April 27, 1955), and Convention Concerning Minimum Age for Admission to Employment (adopted June 26, 1973, 1015 U.N.T.S. 298, entered into force June 19, 1976).

8. Cathy Albisa and Jessica Schultz, "The United States: A Ragged Patchwork," in Social Rights Jurisprudence: Emerging Trends in International and Comparative Law, ed. Malcolm Langford (Cambridge, UK: Cambridge University Press, 2009), 230.

9. Philip Harvey, "Joblessness and the Law before the New Deal," Georgetown Journal on Law and Poverty 6, no. 1 (1999): 11–41. Harvey reviews the English and U.S. poor relief systems. Theda Skocpol, Protecting Soldiers and Mothers: The Political Origins of Social Policy in the United States (Cambridge, MA: Harvard University Press, 1992). Skocpol reviews the social welfare programs for soldiers and their dependents and for mothers and dependent children in the late nineteenth and early twentieth centuries.

10. Michael Hiltzik, The New Deal: A Modern History (New York: Free Press, 2011).

11. Franklin Delano Roosevelt, "Franklin Delano Roosevelt, President, United States of America, State of the Union Message to Congress, January 11, 1944," The American Presidency Project, http://www.presidency.ucsb.edu/ws/index.php?pid=16518. At least one commentator says that Roosevelt's speech may be the greatest of the twentieth century; Lincoln Caplan, "The Legal Olympian: Cass Sunstein and the Modern Regulatory State," Harvard Magazine, January–February 2015, http://harvardmagazine.com/2015/01/the-legal-olympian#.VJSslGlbqR4.email.

12. Franklin Delano Roosevelt, "Franklin Delano Roosevelt, President, United States of America, Annual Message to Congress on the State of the Union, January 6, 1941," The American Presidency Project, http://www.presidency.ucsb.edu/ws/index.php?pid=16092.

13. United Nations, "Constitution of the World Health Organization, U.N. Doc. E/155 (1946)," October 2006, http://www.who.int/governance/eb/who_constitution_bn.pdf; United Nations, "Universal Declaration of Human Rights (UDHR)," G.A. Res. 217A (III) (1948), Art. 25, http://www.un.org/en/documents/udhr/. Portions of this section were originally published as Fran Quigley, "The Trans-Pacific Partnership and Access to Medicines," Health and Human Rights Journal, June 18, 2015, http://www.hhrjournal.org/2015/06/the-trans-pacific-partnership-and-access-to-medicines/.

14. World Health Organization, International Conference on Primary Health Care, Declaration of Alma-Ata, Alma-Ata, U.N. Doc. A56/27 (1978), para. I, September 1978, http://www.who.int/publications/almaata_declaration_bn.pdf.

15. Office of the United Nations Commissioner for Human Rights, "International Covenant on Economic, Social and Cultural Rights (ICESCR)," G.A. Res., 2200A (XXI), Art. 12, December 16, 1966, http://www.ohchr.org/EN/ProfessionalInterest/Pages/CESCR.aspx.

16. United Nations, "Committee on Economic, Social and Cultural Rights, General Comment No. 14, the Right to the Highest Attainable Standard of Health," UN Doc. No. E/C.12/2000/4, August 11, 2000, http://docstore.ohchr.org/SelfServices/FilesHandler.ashx?enc-=4slQ6QSmlBEDzFEovLCuW1AVC1NkPsgUedPlF1vfPMJ2c7ey6PAz2qaojTzDJmC0y%2b9 t%2bsAtGDNzdEqA6SuP2r0w%2f6sVBGTpvTSCbiOr4XVFTqhQY65auTFbQRPWNDxL,- paras. 12, 43(d); World Health Organization, "WHO Model List of Essential Medicines, 19th List," August 2015, http://www.who.int/selection_medicines/committees/expert/20/EML_2015_ FINAL_amended_AUG2015.pdf?ua=1. The Human Rights Council, which is composed of UN member countries and adopts resolutions by vote, has recently confirmed that the right to health includes access to medicines generally, not just medicines on the WHO list; Human Rights Council, "Access to Medicines in the Context of the Right of Everyone to the Enjoyment of the Highest Attainable Standard of Physical and Mental Health," A/HRC/23/L.10/Rev. 1, June 11, 2013. The global community has reached consensus on the United Nations, "Sustainable Development Goals for 2030," 2016, http://www.un.org/sustainabledevelopment/. Although the goals do not have the status of human rights law, they do reflect the worldwide agreement on the importance of access to medicine. Specifically, Goal 3, "Ensure healthy lives and promote well-being for all at all ages," includes among its targets "access to safe, effective, quality and affordable essential medicines and vaccines for all"; a focus on neglected diseases; and compliance with the Doha Declaration that reaffirms TRIPS flexibilities to provide access to medicines for all.

17. National Economic and Social Rights Initiative, "What Is the Human Right to Health and Healthcare?" http://www.nesri.org/programs/what-is-the-human-right-to-health-and-health-care (accessed June 17, 2016).

18. Office of the United Nations High Commissioner for Human Rights and Joint United Nations, "International Programme on HIV/AIDS, HIV/AIDS and Human Rights: International Guidelines: Third International Consultation on HIV/AIDS and Human Rights," July 2002, http://www.ohchr.org/Documents/Publications/HIVAIDSGuidelinesen.pdf, para. 45. See also S. Katrina Perehudoff, Richard O. Laing, and Hans V. Hogerzeil, "Access to Essential Medicines in National Constitutions," Bulletin of the World Health Organization 88, no. 11 (2010): 800, doi: 10.2471/BLT.10.078733.

19. World Health Organization, "Access to Essential Medicines as Part of the Right to Health," 2016, http://www.who.int/medicines/areas/human_rights/en/.

20. Shreerupa Mitra-Jha, "UN Human Rights Council Adopts Landmark Resolution on Access to Medicines," First Post, July 2, 2016, http://www.firstpost.com/world/un-human-rights-council-adopts-landmark-resolution-on-access-to-medicines-2868570.html; Human Rights Council, "Access to Medicines."

21. UN Secretary-General and Co-Chairs of the High-Level Panel, "Final Report: United Nations Secretary-General's High-Level Panel on Access to Health Technologies: Promoting Innovation and Access to Health Technologies," September 14, 2016, 20, http://www.unsgac cessmeds.org/final-report.

22. United Nations Office of the High Commissioner, "International Convention on the Elimination of All Forms of Racial Discrimination," G.A. Res. 2106A (1965), para. 5(e) (iv), http://www.ohchr.org/EN/ProfessionalInterest/Pages/CERD.aspx; United Nations, International Convention on the Elimination of All Forms of Discrimination against Women, G.A. Res. 34/180 (1979), article 11.1 (f) and 12, http://www.un.org/womenwatch/daw/cedaw/ text/econvention.htm; United Nations Office of the High Commissioner, "Convention on the Rights of the Child," G.A. Res. 44/25 (1989), Article 24, http://www.ohchr.org/en/profession

alinterest/pages/crc.aspx; Council or Europe, European Social Charter, 529 U.N.T.S. 89 (1961), Article 11, http://conventions.coe.int/treaty/en/Treaties/Html/163.htm; Organisation of African Unity, African Charter on Human and People's Rights, OAU Doc. No. CAB/LEG/67/3 rev. 5 (1981) Article 16, African Commission on Human and People's Rights, http://www.achpr.org/instruments/achpr/; Organization of American States, Additional Protocol to the American Convention on Human Rights in the Area of Economic, Social and Cultural Rights, (Protocol of San Salvador) (1988), Article 10; http://www.oas.org/juridico/english/treaties/a-52.html; Perehudoff, Laing, and Hogerzeil, "Access to Essential Medicines"; S. Katrina Perehudoff, Brigit Toebes, and Hans V. Hogerzeil, "Essential Medicines in National Constitutions: Progress since 2008." Health and Human Rights Journal 18, no. 1 (2016), https://www.hhrjournal.org/2016/05/essential-medicines-in-national-constitutions-progress-since-2008/?platform=hootsuite. According to Perehudoff, Toebes, and Hogerzeil, twenty-two nations have constitutions that oblige governments to protect and/or to fulfill accessibility of, availability of, and/or quality of medicines.

23. Hans V. Hogerzeil, Melanie Samson, Jaume Vidal Casanovas, and Ladan Rahmani-Ocora, "Is Access to Essential Medicines as Part of the Fulfillment of the Right to Health Enforceable through the Courts?" Lancet 368 (2006): 305–11; Global Health Justice Partnership, A Human Rights Approach to Intellectual Property and Access to Medicines (New Haven: Yale Law School and Yale School of Public Health, 2013), 11–24.

24. United Nations, "Universal Declaration of Human Rights (UDHR)," G.A. Res. 217A (III) (1948), Art. 27(2); "International Covenant on Economic, Social and Cultural Rights (ICESCR)," G.A. Res., 2200A (XXI), Art. 15.

25. Committee on Economic, Social and Cultural Rights, General Comment No. 17, U.N. Doc. E/C.12/GC/1712 (2006), paras 3.5, 1–3, http://docstore.ohchr.org/SelfServices/FilesHandler.ashx?enc=4slQ6QSmlBEDzFEovLCuW1a0Szab0oXTdImnsJZZVQcMZjyZlUmZS43h49u0CNAuJIjwgfzCL8JQ1SHYTZH6jsZteqZOpBtECZh96hyNh%2f%2fHW6g3fYyiDXsSgaAmIP%2bP.

26. United Nations, "Committee on Economic, Social and Cultural Rights, General Comment No. 14," paras. 35, 39; J. G. Ruggie, Special Representative of the Secretary-General on the Issue of Human Rights and Transnational Corporations and Other Business Enterprises, "Guiding Principles on Business and Human Rights: Implementing the United Nations 'Protect, Respect and Remedy' Framework," UN Doc. No. A/HRC/17/31 (2011), para. 9, 12, http://www.ohchr.org/Documents/Issues/Business/A-HRC-17-31_AEV.pdf.

27. Committee on Economic, Social and Cultural Rights, "Statement of the ESCR Committee to the Third Ministerial Conference of the WTO," E/C 12/1999/9 (1999), paras. 5 and 6, http://www.cetim.ch/en/documents/codesc-1999-9-eng.pdf.

28. Anand Grover, "Promotion and Protection of All Human Rights, Civil, Political, Economic, Social and Cultural Rights, Including the Right to Development, Report of the Special Rapporteur on the Right of Everyone to the Enjoyment of the Highest Attainable Standard of Physical and Mental Health," A/HRC/11/12, March 31, 2009, http://www2.ohchr.org/english/bodies/hrcouncil/docs/11session/A.HRC.11.12_bn.pdf, 21–29.

29. "UN Experts Voice Concern Over Adverse Impact of Free Trade and Investment Agreements on Human Rights," Office of the United Nations High Commissioner for Human Rights (June 2, 2015), http://www.ohchr.org/FR/NewsEvents/Pages/DisplayNews.aspx?NewsID=16031&LangID=E. Other UN bodies that have expressed concerns about the human rights implications of TRIPS-Plus agreements include the World Health Organization and UN Millennium Development Goals Gap Task Force. Examples include World Health Organization, Resolution WHA61.21, recommending that member states "take into account . . . the impact on public health when considering adoption or implementing more extensive

intellectual property protection than is required by the Agreement on Trade-Related Aspects of Intellectual Property Rights"; World Health Organization, "Sixty First World Health Assembly," 2006), http://apps.who.int/gb/ebwha/pdf_files/WHA61-REC1/A61_Rec1-part2-en.pdf, 44; World Health Organization Briefing Note for 2006 criticizing data exclusivity and stating that "[TRIPS-PLUS] is a worrying trend . . . countries should therefore be vigilant and should not 'trade away' their people's right to have access to medicines"; World Health Organization, "Briefing Note, Access to Medicines," March, 2006, http://www.wpro.who.int/hiv/documents/docs/BriefingNote2DataexclusivityMarch2006_47A0.pdf?ua=1; The UN Millennium Development Goals Gap Task Force, stating that "Developing countries should carefully assess possible adverse impacts on access to medicines when adopting TRIPS-plus provisions"; United Nations, "Table of Recommendations of the MDG Gap Task Force Report 2012, 'The Global Partnership for Development: Making Rhetoric a Reality,' " 2012, http://www.un.org/en/development/desa/policy/mdg_gap/mdg_gap2012/table_recommendations.pdf.

30. United Nations, "Committee on Economic, Social and Cultural Rights, General Comment No. 14," para. 42; Ruggie, "Guiding Principles," Principle 13.

31. Paul Hunt, "Report of the Special Rapporteur on the Right of Everyone to the Enjoyment of the Highest Attainable Standard of Physical and Mental Health," UN Doc. No. A/63/263 (2008), United Nations, www.who.int/medicines/areas/human_rights/A63_263.pdf.

32. Ibid., 17, 20-22.

Conclusion

1. Portions of this section were originally published as Fran Quigley, "A Bitter Pill: Can Access to Medicine Advocates Score Another Victory?" Foreign Affairs, October 18, 2015, https://www.foreignaffairs.com/articles/south-africa/2015-10-18/bitter-pill.

2. Raymond A. Smith and Patricia D. Siplon, Drugs into Bodies: Global AIDS Treatment Activism (Westport, CT: Praeger, 2006), 42.

3. Ibid., 53.

4. Hiroaki Mitsuya, Kent Weinhold, Robert Yarchoan, Dani Bolognesi, and Samuel Broder, "Credit Government Scientists with Developing Anti-AIDS Drug," Letter to the Editor, New York Times, September 28, 1989, http://www.nytimes.com/1989/09/28/opinion/l-credit-government-scientists-with-developing-anti-aids-drug-015289.html.

5. Smith and Siplon, Drugs into Bodies, x, ix, 59.

6. Ibid.

7. Barton Gellman, "An Unequal Calculus of Life and Death: As Millions Perished in Pandemic, Firms Debated Access to Drugs," Washington Post, December 27, 2000, http://www.washingtonpost.com/wp-dyn/content/article/2006/06/09/AR2006060901287.html.

8. World Health Organization, "AIDS Epidemic Update," December 2001, http://data.unaids.org/publications/irc-pub06/epiupdate01_bn.pdf, 2. For global statistics, see UN AIDS, "HIV with Uncertainty Bounds 1990–2012", 2013, http://www.unaids.org/en/resources/campaigns/globalreport2013/globalreport/. Compare Christopher Murray et al., "Global, Regional, and National Incidence and Mortality for HIV, Tuberculosis, and Malaria during 1990–2013: A Systematic Analysis for the Global Burden of Disease Study 2013," Lancet 384, no. 9947 (2014): 1005–70, doi: 10.1016/S0140-6736(14)60844-8.

9. UN AIDS, "South Africa Fact Sheet," 2004, http://data.unaids.org/Publications/Fact-Sheets01/southafrica_bn.pdf.

10. Treatment Action Campaign, "1998–2010 Fighting for Our Lives: The History of the Treatment Action Campaign," http://www.tac.org.za/files/10yearbook/files/tac%2010%20year%20draft5.pdf, 10.

11. Smith and Siplon, Drugs into Bodies, 62

12. Quoted in Karen DeYoung, "Global AIDS Strategy May Prove Elusive," Washington Post, April 23, 2001, https://www.highbeam.com/publications/the-washington-post-p5554/apr-23-2001.

13. I provide a more detailed account of this scene and of the broader struggle for HIV/AIDS treatment in Kenya and beyond in Fran Quigley, Walking Together, Walking Far: How a U.S.-African Medical School Partnership Is Winning the Fight against HIV/AIDS (Bloomington: Indiana University Press, 2009), 67.

14. Most Kenyans in the Eldoret area have Christian first names and more traditional last names. I changed the names of all the hospital patients I mention here.

15. Treatment Action Campaign, "1998–2010 Fighting for Our Lives"; Christopher J. Colvin and Steven Robins, "Social Movements and HIV/AIDS in South Africa," in HIV/AIDS in South Africa 25 Years On, ed. Poul Rohleder, Leslie Swartz, Seth Kalichman, and Leickness Simbayi (New York: Springer-Verlag, 2009), 155.

16. Ibid., 159.

17. Mark Heywood, "South Africa's Treatment Action Campaign (TAC): An Example of a Successful Human Rights Campaign for Health," in Introduction: Politics, Human Rights and Poor Global Health: Can Campaigns to Prevent and Treat HIV and AIDS Revive and Strengthen Campaigns for the Right to Health, Access to Legal Services and Social Justice? (Johannesburg: Treatment Action Campaign, 2008), chap. 3, http://www.tac.org.za/community/node/2064; Smith and Siplon, Drugs into Bodies, 30.

18. Heywood, "South Africa's Treatment Action Campaign," chap. 3.

19. Ibid., 19.

20. In Anne-Christine D'Adesky and Ann T. Rossetti, Pills, Profits, Protest, [Film], Democracy Now, 2003.

21. Colvin and Robins, "Social Movements," 159.

22. Ibid., 158.

23. Treatment Action Campaign, "1998–2010 Fighting for Our Lives," 20.

24. Ibid., 52.

25. Smith and Siplon, Drugs into Bodies, 85.

26. Treatment Action Campaign, "1998–2010 Fighting for Our Lives," 39.

27. Ibid., 36.

28. Sarah Bosely, "Big Pharma's Worst Nightmare," Guardian, January 26, 2016, http://www.theguardian.com/society/2016/jan/26/big-pharmas-worst-nightmare.

29. Quoted in Smith and Siplon, Drugs into Bodies, 81.

30. Ibid., 98.

31. Ibid., 64.

32. Tina Rosenberg, "Look at Brazil," New York Times, January 28, 2001, http://www.nytimes.com/2001/01/28/magazine/look-at-brazil.html.

33. Quoted in Smith and Siplon, Drugs into Bodies, 105.

34. Ibid., 52–53.

35. Charles R. Babcock and Ceci Connolly, "AIDS Activists Badger Gore Again," Washington Post, June 18, 1999, http://www.washingtonpost.com/wp-srv/politics/campaigns/wh2000/stories/gore061899.htm; Smith and Siplon, Drugs into Bodies, 63–68; "Candidate GORE Zaps," ACT-UP, http://actupny.org/actions/gorezaps.html (accessed June 17, 2016).

36. Smith and Siplon, Drugs into Bodies, 67.

37. Ibid., 102.

38. Ibid., 98–99; "AIDS Drugs for Africa March and Rally," ACT Up, last modified March 5, 2001, http://www.actupny.org/reports/march5.html.

39. Smith and Siplon, Drugs into Bodies, 99; Rachel L. Swairns, "Drug Companies Drop South Africa Suit over AIDS Medicine," New York Times, April 20, 2001, http://www.nytimes.com/2001/04/20/world/drug-makers-drop-south-africa-suit-over-aids-medicine.html. Swairns quotes the CEO of GlaxoSmithKline: "We are not insensitive to public opinion. That is a factor in our decision-making."

40. Smith and Siplon, Drugs into Bodies, 99; John S. James, "March 5: 'Global Day of Action against Drug Company Profiteering,' as Pharmaceutical Companies Sue South Africa to Block Low-Cost Medicines," The Body January 26, 2005, http://www.thebody.com/content/art32009.html; Eduard Grebe, "The Treatment Action Campaign's Struggle for AIDS Treatment in South Africa," Journal of Southern African Studies 37, no. 4 (2011): 849–68, doi: http://dx.doi.org/10.1080/03057070.2011.608271.

41. Smith and Siplon, Drugs into Bodies, 67.

42. World Trade Organization, "Ministerial Declaration of 14 November 2001," WT/MIN(01)/DEC/1, 41 I.L.M. 746 (November 14, 2001), https://www.wto.org/english/thewto_e/minist_e/min01_e/mindecl_trips_e.htm, para. 4.

43. Ellen t'Hoen, The Global Politics of Pharmaceutical Monopoly Power: Drug Patents, Access, Innovation and the Application of the WTO Doha Declaration on TRIPS and Public Health (Diemen, Netherlands: AMB, 2009), 44–62, http://www.msfaccess.org/sites/default/files/MSF_assets/Access/Docs/ACCESS_book_GlobalPolitics_tHoen_BNG_2009.pdf.

44. Smith and Siplon, Drugs into Bodies, 123.

45. Brook Baker, "Placing Access to Essential Medicine on the Human Rights Agenda," in The Power of Pills: Social, Ethical and Legal Issues in Drug Development, Marketing and Pricing 245, ed. Jillian Clare Cohen, Patricia Illingworth, and Udo Schüklenk (Ann Arbor: Pluto Press, 2006).

46. Quigley, Walking Together, Walking Far, 57–59; Smith and Siplon, Drugs into Bodies, 130, 135.

47. Quigley, Walking Together, Walking Far, 56, 62.

48. Brook Baker, "International Collaboration on IP and Access to Medicines: The Birth of the S. Africa Fix the Patents Law Campaign," New York Law School Law Review 60, no. 2 (2015–2016: 297–330).

49. UN AIDS, "World AIDS Day Report 2015," http://www.unaids.org/sites/default/files/media_asset/AIDS_by_the_numbers_2015_bn.pdf.

50. In Fire in the Blood [film], directed by Dylan Mohan Gray, September 7, 2013, Sparkwater India. After antiretrovirals became widely available in South Africa, Achmat finally agreed to take them himself.

51. Peter Drahos and John Braithwaite, "Briefing 32: Who Owns the Knowledge Economy? Political Organising behind TRIPS," The Corner House, September 30, 2004, http://www.thecornerhouse.org.uk/resource/who-owns-knowledge-economy.

52. Brook Baker and Tenu Avafia. "The Evolution of IPRs from Humble Beginnings to the Modern Day TRIPS-Plus Era: Implications for Treatment Access," Working paper, Global Commission on HIV and the Law, UN Development Programme, New York, July 2011, 2

53. D. Singh Grewal and Amy Kapczynski, "Let India Make Cheap Drugs," New York Times, December 11, 2014, http://www.nytimes.com/2014/12/12/opinion/let-india-make-cheap-drugs.html; Médecins Sans Frontières/Doctors Without Borders, Persistent US attacks on India's Patent Law & Generic Competition (New York: MSF, 2015), https://www.msfaccess.org/sites/default/files/IP_US-India_Briefing%20Doc_final_2%20pager.pdf.

54. Ellen t'Hoen, "Access to Cancer Treatment: A Study of Medicine Pricing Issues with Recommendations for Improving Access to Cancer Medication," Oxfam, February 2015, https://www.oxfam.org/sites/www.oxfam.org/files/file_attachments/rr-access-cancer-treatment-inequality-040215-en.pdf, 36.

55. Rupali Mukherjee, "US Pharma Body Slams Indian Patent Regime," Times of India, February 9, 2016, http://timesofindia.indiatimes.com/business/india-business/US-pharma-body-slams-Indian-patent-regime/articleshow/50908408.cms. Mukherjee reports that PhRMA complained that India's "legal and regulatory systems pose procedural and substantive barriers at every step of the patent process."

56. Shreerupa Mitra-Jha, "US Report Puts India on 'Priority Watch List,' Raises Concerns over Pharma Sector," Firstpost, April 29, 2016, http://www.firstpost.com/world/united-states-us-priority-watch-list-ipr-pharma-2756774.html.

57. Sarah Asrar and Fran Quigley, "India's Patent Problems," Foreign Affairs, June 12, 2016, https://www.foreignaffairs.com/articles/india/2016-06-12/indias-patent-problems.

58. Brook K. Baker, "LDCs Be Damned: USTR and Big Pharma Seeks to Eviscerate Least Developed Countries' Insulation from Pharmaceutical Monopolies," InfoJustice.org, October 12, 2015, http://infojustice.org/archives/35147; James Love, "USTR Releases Documents from 2012 R&D Treaty Negotiations," Knowledge Ecology International, September 21, 2015, http://keion line.org/node/2325; Tracy Seipel, "High-Cost Drugs: California Legislator Pulls Bill Seeking Cost Transparency," San Jose Mercury News, January 13, 2016, http://www.mercurynews.com/health/ci_29376102/california-legislator-pulls-bill-that-sought-transparency-high;SarahKarlin-Smithand Brett Norman, "Pharma Campaign against CA Ballot Measure Tops $126M," Politico, November 2, 2016, http://www.politico.com/tipsheets/prescription-pulse/2016/10/pharma-campaign-against-ca-ballot-measure-tops-126mkaiser-consumer-out-of-pocket-drug-spending-fell-through-2014pricing-pressure-leads-to-r-d-changes-217145#ixzz4OmshQbYl.

59. Charles V. Allen, "Despite Misleading Ads, Allowing Drug Negotiations Would Lower Prices," Modesto Bee, April 14, 2016, http://www.modbee.com/opinion/opn-columns-blogs/community-columns/article71872487.html#storylink=cpy.

60. Quoted in Kimberly Leonard, "Budget Breakers: The Increasing Cost of Prescription Drugs Makes Both Families and Governments Go into the Red," U.S. News and World Report, September 24, 2015, http://www.usnews.com/news/the-report/articles/2015/09/24/expensive-drugs-a-drag-on-consumers-and-government.

61. Keith Bradsher and Andrew Pollack, "What Changes Lie Ahead from the Trans-Pacific Partnership Pact," New York Times, October 5, 2015, http://www.nytimes.com/2015/10/06/business/international/what-changes-lie-ahead-from-the-trans-pacific-partnership-pact.html.

62. Deborah Cohen, "Will Industry Influence Derail UN Summit?" BMJ 343: d5328, doi: http://dx.doi.org/10.1136/bmj.d5328; Baker and Avafia, "Evolution of IPRs," 4.

63. Thomas Fuller, "Thailand Takes on Drug Industry, and May Be Winning," New York Times, April 11, 2007, http://www.nytimes.com/2007/04/11/world/asia/11iht-pharma.4.5240 049.html?pagewanted=all.

64. "International NGO Solidarity Statement: US-Thai Free Trade Negotiations Threaten Access to Medicines; Activists Demand Suspension of Negotiations and End to TRIPS-Plus IP Provisions," CPTech, January 9, 2006, http://www.cptech.org/ip/health/c/thailand/solidari tystatement01092006.doc; Smith and Siplon, Drugs into Bodies, 92; t'Hoen, "Access to Cancer Treatment," 19.

65. Julia Paley, "Where the TPP Could Lose: Activists in Chile Have Made Their Government Draw Red Lines on the Corporate-Friendly Investment Deal. North Americans Could Take a Lesson," Foreign Policy in Focus, August 12, 2015, http://fpif.org/where-the-tpp-could-lose/; Andrew Goldman, "Chilean Cámara de Diputados Votes Overwhelmingly to Advance Compulsory Licensing of Drug Patents," Knowledge Ecology International, January 25, 2017, http://keionline.org/node/2716.

66. Baker and Avafia, "Evolution of IPRs."

67. James Love and Andrew S. Goldman, "Colombia Asked to Declare Excessive Price for Cancer Drug Contrary to Public Interest, Grounds for Compulsory License," IPWatch,

December 3, 2015, http://www.ip-watch.org/2015/12/03/colombia-asked-to-declare-excessive-price-for-cancer-drug-contrary-to-public-interest-grounds-for-compulsory-license/; Smith and Siplon, Drugs into Bodies, 90–91.

68. Smith and Siplon, Drugs into Bodies; Global Health Justice Partnership, A Human Rights Approach to Intellectual Property and Access to Medicines (New Haven: Yale Law School and Yale School of Public Health, 2013), 17–18.

69. João Biehl, Mariana P. Socal, and Joseph J. Amon, "The Judicialization of Health and the Quest for State Accountability: Evidence from 1,262 Lawsuits for Access to Medicines in Southern Brazil," Health and Human Rights Journal 18, no. 1 (2016): 209–20, http://www.hhrjournal.org/2016/04/the-judicialization-of-health-and-the-quest-for-state-accountability-evidence-from-1262-lawsuits-for-access-to-medicines-in-southern-brazil/.

70. Portions of this section were drawn from Fran Quigley, "The TPP's Bad Medicine," Foreign Affairs, July 13, 2015, https://www.foreignaffairs.com/articles/2015-07-13/tpps-bad-medicine.

71. Quoted in "Silva: Perú No Cambiará Acuerdos de Patentes con Estados Unidos," Noticias, June 12, 2013, http://rpp.pe/economia/economia/silva-peru-no-cambiara-acuerdos-de-patentes-con-estados-unidos-noticia-603628.

72. Australian Government Department of Foreign Affairs and Trade, "Frequently Asked Questions on Intellectual Property and Public Health Issues," http://dfat.gov.au/trade/agreements/tpp/pages/frequently-asked-questions-on-intellectual-property-and-public-health-issues.aspx (accessed June 17, 2016).

73. Quoted in Noushin Khushushrahi, "Malaysia's PM: More Scrutiny and Flexibility Is Required around the TPP," Open Media, October 8, 2013, https://openmedia.org/en/malaysias-pm-more-scrutiny-and-flexibility-required-around-tpp.

74. Peter Maybarduk, "TPP Chiefs Raise Doubts about USTR's Corporate IP Wish List," Public Citizen, May 30, 2012, http://citizen.typepad.com/eyesontrade/2012/05/tpp-chiefs-raise-doubts.html; New Zealand Labour Party, "Government, Not Wikileaks, Should Reveal Facts about TPP," Scoop, November 14, 2013, http://www.scoop.co.nz/stories/PA1311/S00243/government-not-wikileaks-should-reveal-tpp-facts.htm; Claudio Ruiz, "Heraldo Muñoz, Chilean Minister of Foreign Affairs and TPP: 'If There Is Not an Acceptable Agreement, We Will Not Sign,'" InfoJustice.org, May 26, 2015, http://infojustice.org/archives/34482 MP Don Davies, "NDP Trade Critic Calls for More Transparency in TPP Negotiations," http://infojustice.org/archives/34482; MP Don Davies, "NDP Trade Critic calls for More Transparency in TPP Negotiations," news release, August 28, 2013, http://dondavies.ca/ndp-trade-critic-calls-for-more-transparency-in-tpp-negotiations/.

75. Quigley, "TPP's Bad Medicine"; interviews with author.

76. Michael Grunwald, "Leaked: What's in Obama's Trade Deal," Politico, July 1, 2015, http://www.politico.com/agenda/story/2015/06/tpp-deal-leaked-pharma-000126.

77. James Trimarco, "How a Battle over Affordable Medicine Helped Kill the TPP," Yes Magazine, November 18, 2016, http://www.yesmagazine.org/new-economy/how-a-battle-over-affordable-medicine-helped-kill-the-tpp-20161118.

78. Adam Behsudi and Sarah Karlin, "Obama Delivers TPP Hard Sell to Pharma CEO's," Politico, October 28, 2015, http://lists.keionline.org/pipermail/ip-health_lists.keionline.org/2015-October/005490.html.

79. Jackie Calmes, "Senator Rob Portman to Oppose Pacific Trade Pact," New York Times February 4, 2016, http://www.nytimes.com/2016/02/05/business/international/senator-rob-portman-to-oppose-pacific-trade-pact.html?_r=0.

80. Ylan Q. Mui, "President Trump Signs Order to Withdraw from Trans-Pacific Partnership," Washington Post, January 23, 2017, https://www.washingtonpost.com/news/wonk/wp/2017/01/23/president-trump-signs-order-to-withdraw-from-transpacific-partnership/?utm_term=.0c321ae17a15.

81. Evan Greer, Tom Morello and Evangeline Lilly "The TPP Wasn't Killed by Donald Trump; Our Protests Worked," The Guardian, November 28, 2016, https://www.theguardian. com/commentisfree/2016/nov/28/tpp-protests-mass-opposition-worked-trump-presidency.

82. Trimarco, "How a Battle over Affordable Medicine."

83. Mui, "President Trump Signs Order to Withdraw from Trans-Pacific Partnership."

84. Joseph Stiglitz and Adam Hersh, "The Trans-Pacific Free-Trade Charade," Project Syndicate, October 2, 2015, https://www.project-syndicate.org/commentary/trans-pacific-partner ship-charade-by-joseph-e--stiglitz-and-adam-s--hersh-2015-10#TvXkSbXMpKwUV2k4.99; Jan Schakowsky. Barbara Lee, George Miller, Rosa DeLauro, Michael Michaud, Jim McDermott, Louise Slaughter, John Conyers, Jr., James P. McGovern, Donna Edwards, Keith Ellison, Raul Grijalva, Henry C. Johnson Jr., Richard M. Nolan, Mark Pocan, Steve Cohen, "Letter to the Hon. Michael Froman," Public Citizen, March 14, 2014, http://www.citizen.org/doc uments/congressoinal-letter-to-ustr-on-TPP-and-medicines-march-2014.pdf; "Hillary Clinton Says She Does Not Support Trans-Pacific Partnership," PBS, October 7, 2015, http://www. pbs.org/newshour/rundown/hillary-clinton-says-she-does-not-support-trans-pacific-partner ship/. According to this PBS report, "pharmaceutical companies may have gotten more benefits and patients fewer." Mike Palmedo, "Candidates Clinton and Sanders on Intellectual Property and Access to Medicines in the TPP and Other Trade Agreements," InfoJustice, April 19, 2016, http://infojustice.org/archives/35928.

85. Benjamin Goad, "AARP Warns Trade Deal Could Lock in High Drug Prices," The Hill, October 23, 2013, http://thehill.com/regulation/healthcare/330199-trade-agreement-could-lock-in-high-drug-prices-aarp-warns; Andis Robeznieks, "Trans Pacific Trade Pact May Carry Healthcare Costs," Modern Healthcare, November 5, 2015, http://www.modern healthcare.com/article/20151105/NEWS/151109933.

86. Fran Quigley, "Disgusted with Sky-High Drug Prices, California Voters Take on Big Pharma," Truthout, August 18, 2016, http://www.truth-out.org/news/item/37260-disgusted-with-sky-high-drug-prices-california-voters-take-on-big-pharma.

87. Austin Frakt, Steven D. Pizer, and Roger Feldman, "Should Medicare Adopt the Veterans Health Administration Formulary?" Health Economics, April 2011, http://papers.ssrn. com/sol3/papers.cfm?abstract_id=1809665.

88. Carly Helfand, "Planes, Hearses, and Caravans Dot 'Gilead Greed Kills' Protests from AIDS Foundation," FiercePharma, June 16, 2016, http://www.fiercepharma.com/ pharma/planes-hearses-and-caravans-dot-gilead-greed-kills-protests-from-aids-foundation.

89. Judith Graham, "Medicaid, Private Insurers Begin to Lift Curbs on Pricey Hepatitis C Drugs," Kaiser Health News, July 6, 2016, http://www.healthleadersmedia.com/finance/ medicaid-private-insurers-begin-lift-curbs-pricey-hepatitis-c-drugs.

90. "Anti-Pharma Activists Run Full-Page Ad in Philly Calling Out DNC and RNC on Their 'Buy-Partisan' Support of Drug Corporations," Common Dreams, July 25, 2016, http:// www.commondreams.org/newswire/2016/07/25/anti-pharma-activists-run-full-page-ad-philly-calling-out-dnc-and-rnc-their-buy?utm_campaign=shareaholic&utm_medium=email_ this&utm_source=email.

91. Nathan Borney, "EpiPen Maker to Offer Discounts after Price Hike Firestorm," USA Today, August 26, 2016, http://www.usatoday.com/story/money/2016/08/25/epipen-maker-offer-discounts-after-firestorm/89329122/.

92. Democracy Now,"Video: Protesters Interrupt U.S. Trade Rep at TPP Hearing," YouTube video, 02:01, January 28, 2015, https://www.youtube.com/watch?v=BIw0XSEXPFk; Peter B. Bach, Leonard B. Saltz, and Robert Wittes, "In Cancer Care, Cost Matters," New York Times, October 15, 2012, http://www.nytimes.com/2012/10/15/opinion/a-hospital-says-no-to-an-11000-a-month-cancer-drug.html?_r=0; Indiana University Robert H. McKinney School of Law, "IU McKinney Clinic Plays Key Role in ACLU Suit against FSSA," news release, December 10, 2015, http://mckinneylaw.iu.edu/news/releases/2015/12/iu-mckinney-

clinic-plays-key-role-in-aclu-suit-against-fssa.html; "'Stop Runaway Drug Pricing' Measure Qualifies for San Francisco Ballot, Says the Committee on Fair Drug Pricing (a.k.a. FAIR)," Business Wire, March 1, 2013, http://www.businesswire.com/news/home/20130301006191/ en/%E2%80%98Stop-Runaway-Drug-Pricing%E2%80%99-Measure-Qualifies-San; "Physicians Call for Fairness in Drug Prices, Availability," American Medical Association Wire, November 17, 2015, http://www.ama-assn.org/ama/ama-wire/post/physicians-call-fairness-drug-prices-availability?utm_source=FBPAGE&utm_medium=Social_AMA&utm_term= 281158990&utm_content=other&utm_campaign=article_alert.

93. Daniel J. Stone, "We're All Paying a High Price for Drug Company Profiteering," Los Angeles Times, July 6, 2016, http://www.latimes.com/opinion/op-ed/la-oe-stone-solvadi-drug-pricing-20160705-snap-story.html.

94. Jeff Clawson, "Op-Ed: Exorbitant Drug Prices Are Nothing Short of Evil," Salt Lake Tribune, January 9, 2016, http://www.sltrib.com/opinion/3386827-155/op-ed-exorbitant-drug-prices-are-nothing.

95. "Faith Groups Declare TPP Investment Chapter Unjust and Puts Profit Ahead of People," Network Lobby, news release, March 27, 2015, http://networklobby.org/legislation/FaithStatementtpp_investment_chapter. See also Fran Quigley, "Prescription for Justice: Catholics Must Help Bring Down Barriers Blocking Billions from Lifesaving Medicine," National Catholic Reporter, October 9, 2015, http://ncronline.org/news/peace-justice/prescription-justice-catholics-must-help-bring-down-barriers-blocking-billions; Catherine Ho, "More than 50 Health, Religious and Labor Groups Urge Congress to Reject TPP Trade Deal," Washington Post, April 12, 2016, https://www.washingtonpost.com/news/powerpost/wp/2016/04/12/more-than-50-health-religious-and-labor-groups-urge-congress-to-reject-tpp-trade-deal/.

96. Ed Silverman, "Interfaith Investor Coalition Pushes Shareholder Resolutions on Drug Prices," STAT, October 24, 2016, https://www.statnews.com/pharmalot/2016/10/24/interfaith-coalition-drug-prices/.

97. PFAM, "People of Faith for Access to Medicines," www.pfamrx.org (accessed November 6, 2016).

98. Union for Affordable Cancer Treatment, "Coalition for Affordable T-DM1 Asks the Government to Employ Crown Use Authority to Lower Price of Expensive Cancer Drug," news release, October 1, 2015, http://cancerunion.org/tdm1_press_release.html; Sarah Boseley, "Big Pharma's Worst Nightmare," Guardian, January 26, 2016, http://www.theguardian.com/society/2016/jan/26/big-pharmas-worst-nightmare.

99. Brian Krans, "Massive Trade Pact Could Inflate Global Drug Prices, Restrict Access," Healthline, October 27, 2015, http://www.healthline.com/health-news/massive-trade-pact-could-inflate-global-drug-prices-restrict-access-102715; Lori Wallach, "Cancer Patient Lays Bare the Danger of TPP and the 'Pharma Bro' Problem," The Blog, Huffington Post, February 11, 2016, http://www.huffingtonpost.com/lori-wallach/-cancer-patient-lays-bare_b_9211092.html.

100. Quoted in Public Citizen, "Cancer Patient Disrupts TPP Negotiations Arrested from Hotel Demanding to See the Secret 'Death Sentence Clause,'" news release, September 30, 2015, http://www.commondreams.org/newswire/2015/09/30/cancer-patient-disrupts-tpp-negotiations.

101. "TWN IP and Health: China's Patent Office Invalidated Novartis' Patent on Gleevec," Third World Network, January 27, 2016, http://twn.my/title2/intellectual_property/info.service/2016/ip160102.htm.

102. Quoted in Michael Atkin and Joel Keep, "Hepatitis C Sufferer Imports Life-Saving Drugs from India, Takes on Global Pharmaceutical Company," ABC News, August 20, 2015, http://www.abc.net.au/news/2015-08-20/hepatitis-c-sufferer-imports-life-saving-drugs-from-india/6712990; Huizhong Wu, "India Buyers Club: The New Way for Americans to Buy

Cheap Drugs," CNN Money, June 2, 2016, http://money.cnn.com/2016/06/02/news/india-buyers-club-sofosbuvir-hepatitis/index.html.

103. Reema Nagarajan, "Hepatitis C Cure May Cost as Low as Rs 67k," Times of India, November 29, 2015, http://timesofindia.indiatimes.com/home/science/Hepatitis-C-cure-may-cost-as-low-as-Rs-67k/articleshow/49966218.cms; Sandeep Kishore, Kavitha Kolappa, Jordan D. Jarvis, Paul H. Park, Rachel Belt, Thirukumaran Balasubramaniam, and Rachel Kiddell-Monroe, "Overcoming Obstacles to Enable Access to Medicines for Noncommunicable Diseases in Poor Countries," Health Affairs 34, no. 9 (2015): 1569–77, doi: 10.1377/hlthaff.2015.0375.

104. t'Hoen, "Access to Cancer Treatment," 19–47.

105. Ibid.

106. Marcus Low and Eduard Grebe, "Transnational Mobilisation on Access to Medicines: The Global Movement around the Imatinib Mesylate Case and Its Roots in the AIDS Movement," December 31, 2014, doi: http://dx.doi.org/10.2139/ssrn.2546392.

107. Ibid., 15.

108. t'Hoen, "Access to Cancer Treatment," 36; Rupali Mukherjee, "US Pharma Body Slams Indian Patent Regime," Times of India, February 9, 2016, http://timesofindia.india times.com/business/india-business/US-pharma-body-slams-Indian-patent-regime/articleshow/50908408.cms.

109. Low and Grebe, "Transnational Mobilisation on Access to Medicines."

110. Ibid.

111. Ibid.

112. t'Hoen, "Access to Cancer Treatment," 36.

113. Médicins Sans Frontières/Doctors Without Borders, MSF Access Campaign website, http://www.msfaccess.org/.

114. Médicins Sans Frontières/Doctors Without Borders, "MSF Launches Global Action against Pfizer and GlaxoSmithKline to Cut the Price of the Pneumonia Vaccine," news release, November 12, 2015, http://www.msfaccess.org/about-us/media-room/press-releases/msf-launches-global-action-against-pfizer-and-glaxosmithkline-cut.

115. Médecins Sans Frontières/Doctors Without Borders, "MSF Welcomes Pfizer's Pneumonia Vaccine Price Reduction for Children in Humanitarian Emergencies," November 15, 2016, https://www.msf.org.au/article/project-news/msf-welcomes-pfizer%E2%80%99s-pneu monia-vaccine-price-reduction-children-humanitarian.

116. James Love, "Trans-Pacific Partnership (TPP also Known as the TPP)," Knowledge Ecology International, December 13, 2010, http://www.keionline.org/tpp.

117. Public Citizen, "Access to Medicines," http://www.citizen.org/Page.aspx?pid=4955 (accessed June 17, 2016).

118. Universities Allied for Essential Medicines, "Make Medicines for People, Not Profit," last modified November, 2015, https://uaem.wufoo.com/forms/make-medicines-for-people-not-for-profit/.

119. PFAM, "People of Faith for Access."

120. "Physicians Call for Fairness"; Quigley, "Disgusted."

121. In D'Adesky and Rossetti, Pills, Profits, Protest.

122. Cancer Families for Affordable Medicine, 2017, http://cancerfam.org/ (accessed February 19, 2017).

123. Type 1 International, 2017, https://www.t1international.com/ (accessed February 19, 2017). Patients for Affordable Drugs, www.patientsforaffordabledrugs.org.

124. Public Citizen, "New Report Takes on Obama Administration Defense"; Tami Luhby, ""Yes, 'President Trump' Could Really Kill NAFTA—but It Wouldn't Be Pretty," CNN Money. July 6, 2016, http://money.cnn.com/2016/07/06/news/economy/trump-nafta/.

125. Bianca DiJulio, Jamie Firth, and Mollyann Brodie, "Kaiser Health Tracking Poll: August 2015," Kaiser Family Foundation, August 20, 2015, http://kff.org/health-costs/poll-finding/kaiser-health-tracking-poll-august-2015/.

126. Fran Quigley, "Growing Political Will from the Grassroots: How Social Movement Principles Can Reverse the Dismal Legacy of Rule of Law Interventions," Columbia Human Rights Law Review 41, no. 13 (2009): 51–52.

127. Dean Baker, "Prescription Drugs and the Trans-Pacific Partnership: Big Pharma Hit by Skills Shortage," Beat the Press, Center for Economic and Policy Research, March 26, 2016, http://cepr.net/blogs/beat-the-press/prescription-drugs-and-the-trans-pacific-partnership-big-pharma-hit-by-skills-shortage.

128. The Campaign for Sustainable Rx Pricing includes longtime medicine access advocates such as the AIDS Healthcare Foundation alongside major insurance companies and even Walmart; The Campaign for Sustainable Rx Pricing, "Who We Are," http://www.csrxp.org/about-the-campaign/ (accessed November 6, 2016). See also Adam Rubenfire, "Drug Price Hikes May Be Hitting Hospitals Harder than Consumers," Modern Healthcare, October 11, 2016, http://www.modernhealthcare.com/article/20161011/NEWS/161019988/drug-price-hikes-may-be-hitting-hospitals-harder-than-consumers.

INDEX

North American Free Trade Agreement
(NAFTA), 116, 121
*Northwestern Journal of Technology and
Intellectual Property*, 80
Novartis, 33, 39–40, 52, 54–55, 76, 111,
166–167
Novo Nordisk, 14

Obama, Barack, 30, 78, 121,
134–135, 163
Onion, The, 24
open-source research for medicines, 85,
170–171
open-source software, 85
opioid analgesics, 22
Orphan Drug Act, U.S., 140–141
Otsuka, 62
Oxfam, 143

pacilatexel (Taxol), 93
parallel importation, 127, 129
Paris Convention of 1833, 104
patent linkage, 3, 79–80
patent thickets, 79–80
patents: and innovation, 83–85, 133,
142–143
   See also compulsory licenses;
   evergreening; parallel importation;
   patents on prescription medicines
Patents and Trademark Amendments Act
(Bayh-Dole Act of 1980), 92–93,
106–107, 129–132
patents on prescription medicines,
13, 73–77, 79–81, 83–85, 136,
142–143
   See also compulsory licenses;
   evergreening; parallel importation
patient advocacy groups, 29–30, 165–168
Patients for Affordable Drugs, 169
pay for delay, 80–81
People of Faith for Access to Medicines
(PFAM), 165, 168
PEPFAR (U.S. President's Emergency Plan
for AIDS Relief), 100, 116, 132, 159
Peru, 162
Pfizer, 21, 24, 26, 31–32, 43–44,
52–53, 55–56, 61–62, 66–67,

105–106, 108, 115, 156–157,
167
"Pharma Bro." *See* Shkreli, Martin
pharmaceutical industry
   CEO pay, 67
   "disease mongering," 53–54
   fraudulent activities, citations for,
   51–53
   involvement in medical education and
   research reporting, 48–51
   lack of incentive to develop drugs for
   the poor, 24, 31–34
   litigation against the South African
   government, 157–158
   lobbying and political contributions,
   13, 71–72, 81, 92, 106–108, 110,
   134–135, 159–161, 169
   marketing costs and strategies, 43–45,
   53–54, 140, 142, 171
   off-label promotion, 52–53
   patient advocacy group funding,
   29–30
   patient assistance programs, 54–55, 72
   pricing strategies, 26, 57–63
   profitability, 65–67
   regulation of, 136 (*see also* Food and
   Drug Administration, U.S.)
   research and development investments,
   37–41, 67, 171
   stock buybacks, 66–67
   tax avoidance, 55–56
   tax deductions, 136
   unpopularity, 48
   See also Pharmaceutical Researchers
   and Manufacturers Association
   (PhRMA); *names of individual
   pharmaceutical companies*
Pharmaceutical Management Agency,
New Zealand (PHARMAC), 135
Pharmaceutical Researchers and
Manufacturers Association
(PhRMA), 8, 37, 57–58, 66, 71–72,
106, 110, 160, 165
Pharmasset, 41, 60
PhRMA. *See* Pharmaceutical Researchers
and Manufacturers Association
Physician Payment Sunshine Act, 48

CPSIA information can be obtained
at www.ICGtesting.com
Printed in the USA
LVOW03s2127051017
551326LV00004B/405/

3119202135889

9 781501 713750